Seeing The Light

Short Stories by
Rick Williams

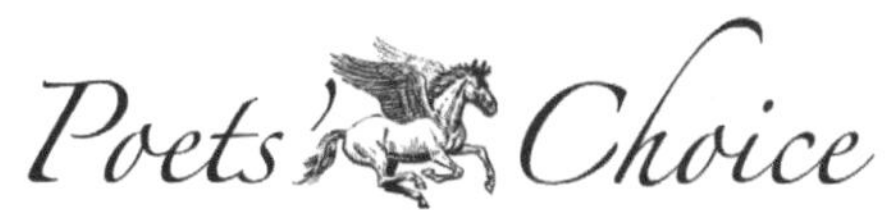

Poets' Choice Publishing

Graphic Design by: Sanket Patel
Paintings by: Rick Williams

Printed in the United States of America
Library of Congress Cataloging-in-Publication Data Pending

ISBN # 978-1-7335400-8-7

About the Cover:

Alvin Sabulsky

WW II, participated in the liberation
of the Dachau Concentration Camp;
Private collection

By Rick Williams

Poets' Choice

Poets' Choice Publishing
337 Kitemaug Road
Uncasville, CT 06382
Poets-Choice.com
marathonfilm@gmail.com

Fourth Edition

Acknowledgment

- Alvin Sabulsky, WW II, participated in the liberation of the Dachau Concentration Camp; private collection
- Wilfredo, KIA, Iraq, age 21; Buffalo VA Regional Office

- Tammy, Iraq; NYC VA Regional Office Museum

- Rick Pringle, Vietnam; private collection

- Vernon Williams; NYC VA Regional Office Museum

- Charles, Vietnam; NYC VA Regional Office Museum

- Joe, Vietnam; NYC VA Regional Office Museum

- Richard Harteis, Portrait by Rick Williams, Private Collection

- Mike Duggan, Vietnam; private collection

- Carl, KIA, Vietnam, age 22; Buffalo VA Regional Office

- Tubie, Vietnam; private collection

- James Carloni, KIA, Vietnam, age 19; private collection

- Tom Mulligan, Vietnam; private collection

- James Mulligan, KIA, WW II, Bougainville, age 26; private collection
- Roy, KIA, WW II; NYC VA Regional Office Museum

- Carlos, KIA, WW II; NYC VA Regional Office Museum

- Rick Williams, Vietnam

- David, KIA, Battle of the Bulge, WW II, age 28, private collection

- Lee, WW II, Buffalo VA Regional Office

- Hue 1968, The Inferno

- "Honor, Valor, Sacrifice, Service" exhibit held in Buffalo VA Regional Office in June 2007
- "Twelve Veterans and their Stories" exhibit held at the NYC VA Regional Office Museum in November 2006

KIA=Killed in action

Aside from active military servicemen killed in action, many of the veterans listed above sustained serious shell fragment and gunshot wounds in combat.

Contents

Introduction

by Richard Harteis

In a previous iteration of this book, the author titled the collection INFINITELY COMPLEX featuring the human brain in a day-glow blue cover. The subtitle read, "Short stories of the ravages of alcoholism and addiction, mental illness, bigotry and (stories of) veterans of war." It is a remarkable collection of broken characters, overwhelmed by spiritual and physical challenges. The new title, SEEING THE LIGHT has as its cover a beautiful portrait of a young soldier who's face is illuminated with inspiration and human compassion. It could be the face of the young medic in the first story of the book, "The Girl in the Oxygen Tent." The boy is disenchanted with the senseless war in Vietnam and finds solace in his love for the young girl who has become his patient. It is a careful description of the Vietnamese culture and the soldier's coming to terms with the pointlessness of this war. When his patient dies, he attends the funeral at some personal risk, and the story simply ends it seems, with no resolution. Like the war itself, there is no answer to the senselessness of death, and the death his country is inflicting on this culture. Many of Rick's stories seem to end this way. He seems to be saying there is nothing to be done in the face of such absurdity. At one point in an email, the author writes that none of the characters in his stories see the light. But the lucky thing for a reader is that he has written these stories and has seen the light through his talent as a storyteller. His is a hard won insight into the ravages he describes. And it takes no little amount of courage to put his experience into these stories. One thinks of the recent autobiography by President Biden's son describing his addiction. Clearly some of the stories are highly autobiographical.

Like many beginning writers, at one point I wrote a novel about my experience in the Peace Corps written in the first person. My friend William Meredith said I could get artistic distance by telling the story in the third person. He even offered to rewrite the book for me. (Had I taken him up on the offer, the book might have ultimately found its way to a publisher.) The "I" in the story was a persona, I tried to explain, was not really me. But it seems clear that Rick's stories are based, in part, on his own struggles. They are simply too actual, too real to be otherwise.

The sole exception to this critique, however, is the excruciating short novella which ends the collection: "A Cunning Baffling Progressive Disease." The protagonist has entered an alcoholism treatment program to avoid divorce by his wife. Throughout the sections of this novella, the central character treats his encounter with a therapist as a kind of boxing match or a game of one ups-manship. He attempts to convince the therapist that he can be a functional alcoholic if he puts in place certain strategies including Ativan to avoid delirium tremens and possible death from alcohol overdose, hiring a big man, a bodyguard to follow him around on his binges and so forth. It is a staggering story of denial and rationalization that must be common in such programs. The therapist, Oscar, proves to be prophetic, and I will not spoil the fantastic dénouement by describing the end of the story. Needless to say, the protagonist hits bottom before events turn about as tragic as one can imagine.

The main character Freddie in this novella is unnerving. He dresses in a white tuxedo like Rick in Casablanca looking for "fellowship with kindred spirits," but this is Rick of Buffalo pub crawling the dives of a working-class neighborhood. The narrator is so full of rationalizations you want to slap him around a bit. It is not easy to listen to him tell his stories with pride and humor. But by the end, one does feel compassion for his hitting bottom as a human being, always remembering how difficult it is to take a long hard look at oneself when you are least attractive. One thinks of Tolstoy's "Death Ivan Ilyich," and the courage it took Tolstoy to write of a man who realizes as he lies dying, that his life has meant nothing; but who, by the end, achieves insight and spiritual awakening.

The collection includes stories which deal all the themes the author outlines, and the techniques he uses to tell the stories are at times a kind of magic realism ("The Illegal Veteran" and "Ciao Jackie Jacko" where the protagonist is a back-up pianist for Frank Sinatra.) Sometimes the stories Incorporate dream, which would be appropriate for an alcoholic who has blacked out and cannot describe what has gone on, why he is in a hotel room with no money and an empty wallet after inviting a woman to his room for a drink. Often, the stories end with no explanation, Beckett like, with mysterious, ominous characters waiting silently, like fate for no particular reason (An Everyday Incident That Chips Away At the Spirit.)

Other stories have a more traditional structure with a beginning middle and end. In "Why Was Jesus Laughing," the brother of a suicide-by-heroin takes it on himself to steal his mother's portrait of Jesus.

Christ's head is actually thrown back in agony. But "salvation is a lie," the narrator explains, and this is why Jesus is "laughing." Human foibles run throughout the story. The frustrated tourist cannot understand why his camera is not working until an innocent bystander points out a piece of gum is covering the camera lens. In another, the protagonist spends his whole life dreaming of his first love and decides to take action and find her. When he finally tracks down an address where she might be, he realizes like a "pensé sur l'escalier," that for all those years he never made any decision to find her. We have all kicked ourselves from time to time at lost opportunity and the paralysis of inaction. Why, why, we ask. But there is no answer. Some of the stories deal with war, but the beautiful portraits throughout this book are not meant to be illustrations of a particular branch of the service or moment in the war. They are there simply to highlight the additional talent the author has a visual artist. These are stunning paintings with great psychological realism and have achieved recognition in museums and private collections throughout the US. Some of the titles of these stories give too much information; the narrator occasionally rolls his eyes too often to show his frustration.

But essentially the stories are there, are clean, are moving, despite the difficult subject matter and the lives of the characters he portrays. We congratulate Rick Williams for this debut collection, and thank him as many veterans have done for his work as a lawyer in their defense as well as the model of compassion and honesty he gives us in the lives of his characters.

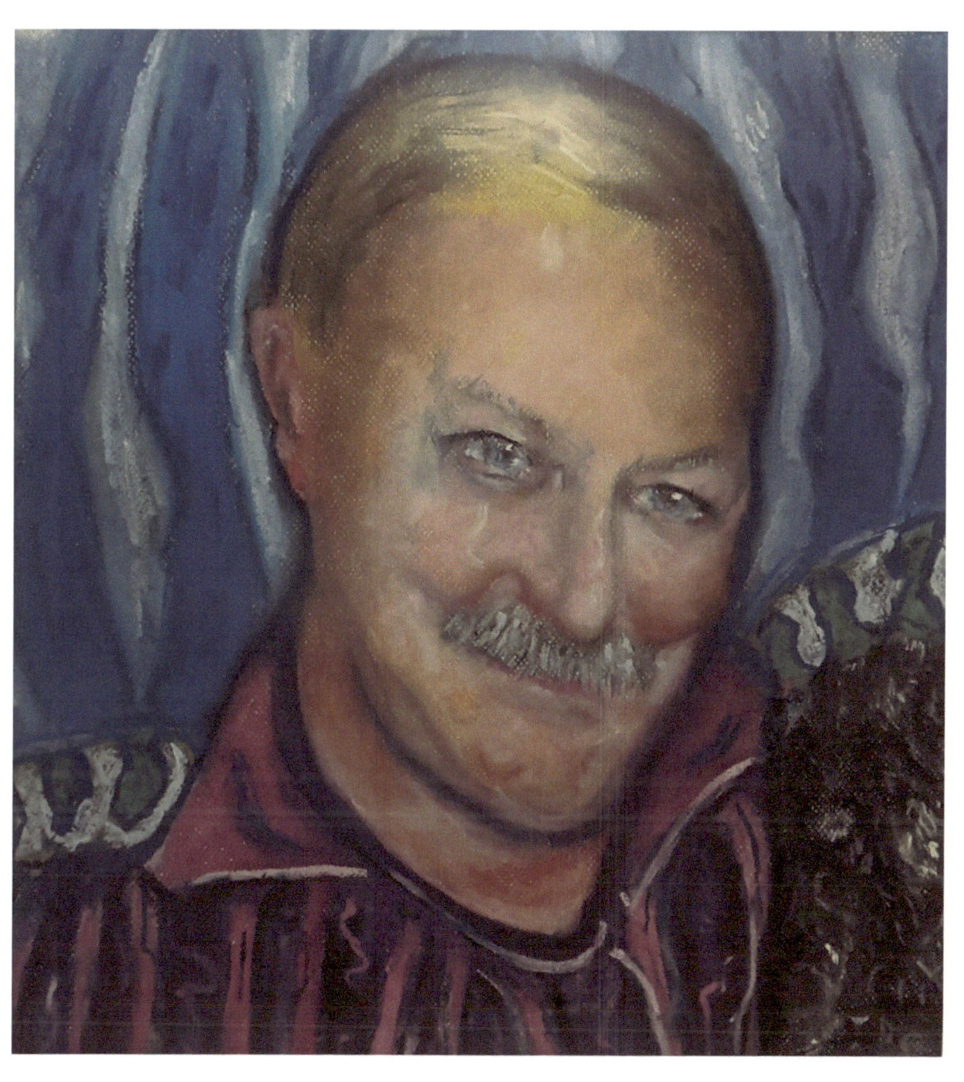

Richard Harteis
Portrait by Rick Williams
Private Collection

Seeing The Light

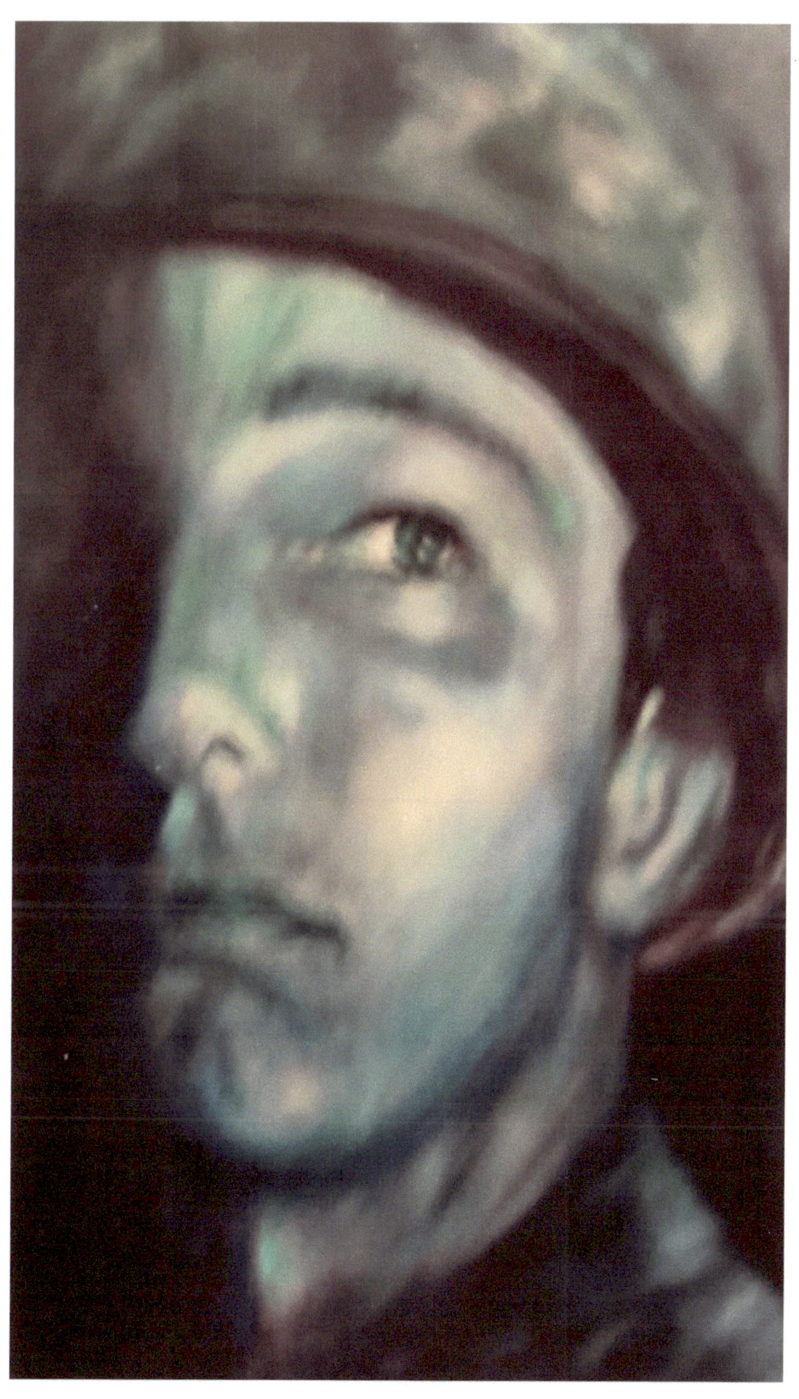

Tubie
Vietnam
Private Collection

The Girl in the Oxygen Tent

While gently peeling off a blood-soaked bandage glued to an above-the-knee stump, I paused and looked at the hazy image. Among all of the torn and burned male bodies, Lan's rectangular space seemed to be of a different world. Stiffly upright and blurred behind plastic walls, it looked like the girl was floating on a carpet that would soon fly away. She was pretty with soft, unblemished skin; high cheekbones; and stoic eyes. But I sensed an undue amount of knowledge and sorrow to burden a pubescent girl. Lan's lips formed a natural pout, but her head seemed too big for her slight body. Always seated while awake, dressed in powder blue pajamas with orange-stripped tigers, her long black hair fell straight to the bed. Her hands were small with barely discernible fingernails.

We bonded primarily through our frequent mutual English and Vietnamese lessons during lulls in the action and when Lan wasn't in respiratory distress. She learned faster than I did. Whether anyone understood our accents outside of the tent was of no matter. We understood each other. And I was able to make her laugh. I often came in on my days off to visit her, and her face would brighten to the extent that was possible. I gave her a large Panda Bear that I bought in the street market. Lan clung to it when she slept.

As the days went by there were more frequent episodes of life-threatening shortness of breath with loud wheezing. During a remission, Lan, with a sheepish expression, asked, "Mr. Lay, can bring me when you go home?"

I answered in English, "I don't think so Lan. It's too far away. Why do you want to leave your home?"

She looked into my eyes and sadly said, "So I can live. I think I die here. I want you take care of me."

I wanted to take care of her, but I wasn't sure why. I didn't know much about myself at age 19.

I began my twelve-hour shift noticing that Lan's bed had been moved closer to the nursing station. She lay in-between a white body cast and a bilateral, above-the-knee amputee—the former a narcotic-induced, sleeping American soldier with multiple fractures of the spine and the latter a post-operative, weeping boy. Despite the continuous flow of oxygen through the tubes in her nose, Lan's respirations were more labored that day. With tightening facial muscles and hands balled up in fists, she tried to speak but could not utter more than a whispered, "No talk now."

Lan managed a weak grin when I tried to pronounce her name. I could not initiate the L sound from the back of my throat no matter how hard I tried. She couldn't pronounce the R of Ray very well either. I lifted the plastic wall to give her a fashion magazine, but Lan's tiny left hand wearily dropped it on the bed. All the doctors and nurses called her Baby San. That's what they called all the Vietnamese girls.

As I tipped and rolled a tall, green oxygen tank toward Lan, I could see apprehension in her eyes. She was taking quick sips of air. I lifted the plastic of her tent to position the heavy tank next to the head of her bed. Lan was so delicate and fragile; I was afraid she would break like a dry twig. I gently put my hand on her shoulder. My presence seemed to alleviate some of her anxiety, but relief was fleeting. The wheezing was louder on that day, evolving into a death moan.

An old woman was allowed to keep vigil. After combing her granddaughter's hair while softly singing in her ear, she emerged from the tent and returned to her position on the floor, cross-legged with a downward gaze under her straw-colored, conical hat. As she looked up, I studied her face with deep furrows that ran like tributaries of a river through sagging flesh. As she looked down to the worn, fading yellow cloth satchel in her lap, she was whispering something. I thought she was praying. I did not know her name. We called all of the old Vietnamese women Mama San.

I was irrigating a deep wound in a young man's abdomen; the bloody liquid was dripping into a narrow, curved silver pan when I turned my head to a high-pitched, agitated noise. The old woman was lifting up her granddaughter's plastic wall with her right hand and waving to me with her downturned left hand, shouting,
"Bác śi. Bác śi." There was urgency in her voice. Bác śi means doctor. I was only a medic.

I took off my sterile plastic gloves and after they dropped to the floor, I put my right hand on the old woman's shoulder, and more firmly placed my left hand on her forearm. I wanted to pull her away carefully from under the oxygen tent as her right hand was under the girl's head. But her arm stiffened and with her left index finger pointing up, she screamed, "Nâng lên! I went to the other side of the bed. Lan was supine with her eyes fixed on the ceiling, and her mouth was sucking air like a fish out of water.

I was inside the plastic tent, pulling the head of the bed up to a 70-degree angle, and I placed two pillows between Lan's back and the bed while yelling for help. Her eyes were big circles looking straight ahead—they never moved—and she began rhythmically sipping more air, but in looking at the movements of her chest, I saw rapid and shallow respirations and her lips were blue. She was suffocating. After giving an inhalant that opened up Lan's airways, the nurse left the tent. Lan was breathing better, but her eyes were still wide with fear.

The old lady slowly picked up each of the contents of her bag, to include clothes and photographs scattered on top of her granddaughter's bed, and she methodically put them back into her satchel. She resumed her seated position on the floor. The old woman's black pajamas had holes in the knees, and the black silk bunched up above her ankles revealed deformed, dirty feet. She looked up and said through rotting and missing teeth, "Gooood Bác śi."

Minutes later, I looked at Lan's gaunt face and asked, "Is that better?" in Vietnamese. She nodded but only slightly; her sliver of a body was limp from fighting for every breath. But she suddenly became rigid with eyes fixed forward. The grandmother caressed Lan's face while singing something in her ear—I thought it was a nursery rhyme—and the terror slowly left Lan's eyes, leaving a wilted body in its wake. The old woman withdrew, turned, and held my left hand with both of her hands and said, "Dep wa." She said I had pretty hands. "You no work." I looked at her wrinkled, deformed hands. Bagging groceries was not exactly manual labor, nor was zipping up body bags.

The two rows of beds in the bright white, rectangular room were filled with men, all young; a boy soldier; and a dying toddler with third degree burns. There were more Vietnamese than Americans as we were withdrawing from the Mekong Delta.

I remember the constant droning of standing fans blowing hot air and collarless blue surgical tops serving as pajamas and cries of anguish and blurs of green fatigues and black boots streaking by. There were tubes coming out of chests and noses and bags of urine and silver bedpans and the smell of Betadine and wounds with thick flaps of flesh and blood. And there was Lan, alone, floating, of a different world.

I got drunk that night. There were two Vietnamese bar maids on duty with long black hair and perpetual smiles. They wore traditional silk dresses called Ao Dai, slit from the waist on both sides revealing silk pants. Tuba's dress was dark blue over white pants. Miss Fe wore bright orange, and I saw black silk through the long triangular opening of her dress.

Miss Fe was petite and pretty. She moved from table to table without making eye contact, going back and forth from the bar with beer cans, sensually moving inside her silk. As she stood at the bar waiting for another tray full of beers, I asked her to be my girlfriend. With her head bowed by shyness, she softly said, "No can do."

From behind the bar, Tuba overheard my plea and said through laughter, "Hey Lay. Too much beer Lay!" She was raunchy, laughed loud, and looked you in the eye without restraint. No one put Miss before Tuba. I would have loved to go out drinking with her.

I wondered how a Vietnamese girl with asthma ended up in the intensive care unit full of broken bodies of men and boys. How utterly terrifying it must be to struggle for every mouthful of air. I wanted to save her.

Greg Monaco, a medic from the ER, sat on the bar stool next to me. Greg, a tall, skinny guy with a mop of curly black hair; a thick, black fu Manchu; and big eyes, perpetually at half mast, asked, "What's happening Ray?"

I answered without turning my head, "Lan's still fighting for her life. If I could, I would bring her home."

"A little young don't you think?" he said with a smirk.

Looking at Tuba wise-cracking her way up and down the bar, I said, "There's nothing sexual about it."

"No? Ever read Lolita?"

Shaking my head no, I answered, "I think I'm drawn to her vulnerability, her helplessness. I'm thinking of coming back as a civilian."

"To take care of her? You're full of shit," Monaco guffawed.

"I wrote to the Swedish Hospital in Saigon. But they want doctors and nurses—not medics.

"Ah! So it's not just Lan. You're feeling guilty, like we're doing something horrible here."

"Maybe. But I'm also drawn to the culture. The importance of duty, loyalty, respect for family. My family's falling apart."

With a raised voice, Monaco cried, "Who are you trying to bullshit? I think it's the women. No wooing necessary here. And all the dope. Or maybe you want to be a hero. But here heroes aren't possible. Not us to them."

Monaco stood up and shouted on his way to take a piss, "All I know is,

I wanna get the fuck out of here."

Walking into the unit the following morning, I gasped when I saw a body wrapped in a white sheet. It was Lan's bed. The old lady stood next to her dead grandchild. She looked up at me and then bowed her head, softly crying while fingering the edge of her cloth satchel. I tenderly touched Lan's shoulder with my fingertips, silently saying a simple Buddhist prayer she had taught me.

I wheeled a gurney into the unit. The old lady put the satchel on her granddaughter's chest, and when a nurse tried to remove it, the old woman forcefully pulled the satchel and put it back. No one tried to remove it after that.

Lan couldn't have weighed more than 60 pounds. The grandmother walked by the side of the gurney as I pushed it out of the unit through the double door. I looked down at the old woman's heavily callused, purple and black-splotched feet. I wondered how she could walk on hot cement with nothing on her feet.

With her tremulous right hand, the old lady put an X on a hospital form at the front desk. I watched through an open door as she took her granddaughter in a cyclo driven by an old, toothless man with the same straw-colored, conical hat, only his was coming apart at the seams. The body was wrapped in a yellow and red striped cloth and laid horizontally on the grandmother's lap.

Still standing in the doorway, I stared at the old man mechanically going up and down like a piston, and the triangular vehicle went down the road, almost disappearing in the shimmering heat. An MP in a helmet took a long time unwrapping the body. I heard the old lady squawking. I wondered how she was able to take her granddaughter's body out, wrapped in South Vietnamese flag. Who was Lan? The grandmother looked 80, but she was probably no older than 50. The cyclo driver must have been close to 80; otherwise, he would have been in the bush fighting on one side or the other.

At the end of my shift, I went to the mess hall, but I had no appetite. The food was always shitty anyway.

Lew Raskin sat across from me. He was a short, chubby guy with thinning dark brown hair behind a receding hairline. Lew was a young lieutenant and a pothead. He was as comfortable mixing with us peons as the brass. He had a graduate degree from someplace—most of us barely got out of high school if that. Raskin wasn't a nurse or doc; I'm not sure what he did. But I remember what he said.

"How's the chopper pilot doing?" Raskin asked while dousing his powdered eggs with hot sauce.

"He died Tuesday. He was only 19."

With his bushy brown eyebrows raised above his black-rimmed, thick glasses, he incredulously asked, "Of a gunshot wound of the leg?"

"Lower leg. But it shattered the tibia and fibula. He died of a blood clot to the lung. He knew he was going to lose the leg, but he told me, 'At least I'm going to get the fuck out of here.' No more than an hour later, he was gasping for air."

Shaking his head, Raskin whispered, "19 years old. And for what?"

"What do you mean for what?"

Raskin looked into my eyes and said, "What the fuck are we doing here? We hear the boom, boom, boom, and feel the vibrations night after night. B-52s must be taking out entire villages. The whole fucking war is one big My Lai."

Thinking of Lan, I asked, "Why do so many of us call girls baby san? Even adult women. They have names."

Raskin stared into his coffee. "It's easier if they don't have to remember names."

"But Lan had a name. She had the same feelings that I do. Some of us think all Vietnamese are the enemy. Yesterday, after Monaco gave the old papa san with a limp some shit, I was glad the chaplain pointed his finger in his face while saying, 'He's on our side.' Maybe I would see them differently if I were getting shot at rather than seeing all the suffering. I don't know." We both got up.

The next day, Miss Tam, a Vietnamese Operating Room nurse I had befriended, came into the unit and gave me a note: Lan Phong Dam, 1259 Binh Thuy, Can Tao. Monday 12. The nurse said, "Lan funeral. You come."

The following morning, I took a cyclo down the main highway for several miles. The driver, another toothless old man with a faded, chewed up blue New York Yankee hat stopped before a grey concrete bridge over one of a hundred tributaries off the wide Mekong River. While rapidly gumming, he pointed to the dirt path that ran along the river and said, "You go." After I paid him, he lingered, mumbling something.

The muddy river and thick jungle with a path in-between lay before me. The path was hard mud and I could hear women rapidly chattering on the other side of the vegetation. I was soaked in sweat. I heard a continuous buzzing sound in the thick bush and had a throbbing sensation in my throat as I realized something could come crawling out of there and bite or sting me dead. As I passed by two boys fishing with tree branches for poles, I stopped abruptly as a rat the size of a big cat ran out of the jungle, across the path, and down the wet muddy embankment with a long, thin tail slithering behind it.

I finally saw a clearing and some huts around a slight right bend of the river. I stopped. The nearest hut looked like it was made of bamboo and tin cans that had been flattened; I could see repeating patterns of red, white, and blue and the words Pabst Blue Ribbon and Coke-a-Cola were overlapping. There was a group of five old men in crisp white shirts; three wore long, thin black ties and all but one were smoking. I paused and took my cap off and ran my right hand with fingers extended from my forehead through my drenched hair several times. The humidity was suffocating. I wondered how people could live in such heat. They didn't seem to sweat.

Three old women, dressed in familiar loose fitting, white cotton blouses and black silk pants, carrying what looked like heavy pots entered the hut, one after the other. I smelled nuoc mam, which is a fish sauce with an odor like a decomposed body, but it magically makes food taste better if you can get past the initial stink.

I looked at my elongated shadow stretching from boots to cap. Streams of sweat were rolling down my back. All of the men looked at me while chattering rapidly, but upon my prolonged gaze, they quickly turned away. Familiar sounds, like a marimba: mo, hi, ba, bo—up, down, up, down— it was hard for me to believe such strange sounds conveyed the same thoughts and feelings that we had.

A canoe glided past in the muddy water, overflowing with green and yellow produce surrounding an old man and two boys. The squatting boys were laughing at me, and the standing old man yelled something while pointing at his cargo, apparently trying to sell me something. I turned around, wanting to disappear.

I suddenly thought about the Viet Cong. My body tensed as I remembered a door gunner saying, "The VC can waltz into any Mekong Delta town whenever they want. It's where they grew up." He clinched his fists. "Hearts and minds my ass."

I lit a cigarette and watched a woman walk out of the hut, purposely swinging her arms in a long arc. She wore a white Ao Dai with white pants under the slit, white gloves that went to her elbows, and large, dark sun glasses. Some of the men said something to her and she cursed them while walking out of my view. She was taller than the men with black hair down to her waist.

Wearing white silk that sparkled in the sun, she could have been walking down some grand boulevard. Even though her fashionable sunglasses covered her eyes, I knew she was beautiful.

Standing awkwardly tall and pale, conspicuously dressed in olive green fatigues, I took my Army cap off and pushed the beak of it into my back pocket. I kept wiping off the sweat that was continuously rolling down my forehead with the large sleeve of my fatigues.

I stood behind two rows of silent people of all ages. I felt a wave of panic because of what they might think of me. I was on the edge of a place I did not belong, intruding on something sacred.

I was able to see over everyone in front of me and as my eyes scanned the circle, I saw at least thirty women and many young girls. There were far fewer males: the five old men and a few small boys. The rest were fighting or dead.

Miss Tam, the Vietnamese nurse came out of the circle and walked over to my right side. I bent down as she whispered while pointing between standing figures, "You see body. Dat Lan on table. Dey wash an make clean. Dat mother."

She was pointing to the elegant woman in white silk standing at the foot of her daughter. Lan was still wrapped in the yellow and red stripped cloth, but I could see her face. Her eyes were closed. It looked like there was white powder on her forehead and cheeks. There was a chopstick between her teeth. The nurse stood on her toes while looking up at me and said, "Dey put rice an money in mouth."

A monk in an orange robe, bare right shoulder, and shaved head walked through an opening in the circle. He stood over Lan's head. Putting his palms and extended fingers together, he prayed out loud. There was no other sound. I watched the mother. She touched the casket but did not shed a tear. I thought of Jackie Kennedy. Was it grace or shock? Or were her feelings dead from too much exposure to a never-ending war.

After the monk stopped his prayers and moved back into the circle, the dead body was placed in a simple, sand colored wood coffin. The cloth remained under Lan in repose. There was stillness until the grandmother started to shake and sob, and she turned to her daughter and wrapped her arms around her, but Lan's mother stood stiffly; her arms hung limp and never moved. I heard wailing from other women and children. Four of the old men looked down at the ground or into the jungle; one was quietly weeping. Besides the nurse, no one paid any attention to me.

While pointing at several people wearing what looked like white turbans, the nurse said, "Family. Bother. Sister. Family." The old woman emptied the contents from her threadbare, yellow cloth satchel, one item at a time, into the coffin. It looked like the same things that spilled all over Lan's death bed. There was much weeping now. I thought of Westmoreland's asinine remark about the Vietnamese, "not valuing human life like us." There was a slight breeze, but it only blew sticky, hot air. I couldn't breathe.

The men came forward and with one at each corner, they lifted the coffin above their shoulders and began to mechanically carry it down a path through the thick, dark green and brown vegetation with flickering rays of light. The monk in billowing orange followed the men with the raised coffin, his hands remaining in prayer, and everyone fell into line behind the monk. I was the second from the last person in the procession; the nurse was behind me. The path opened up to another large clearing, and there was a rectangular hole in the ground. The men carefully laid the coffin next to the freshly dug hole—large piles of dirt were on each side of the grave—and then they merged into what was now the same circle except for the monk, grandmother, and mother. The latter three were standing on the near side of the coffin with their backs to me. The old woman put another photograph in the coffin for her granddaughter's journey.

Suddenly, I heard the heavy thump-thump sound of a helicopter and as it got louder, most of us looked up to see a Chinook, a huge American helicopter with a distinctive loud thumping sound coming from its two big blades. Inexplicably, the massive helicopter lowered and menacingly hovered for minutes that seemed like an eternity. It was such an intrusive sound. It finally flew up and out of sight, its thumping only slowly fading away.

Some in the circle began lighting what looked like paper objects and dropping them near the coffin. The slight breeze brought a pleasant smell of incense. The four pallbearers came out of the circle; two of them lifted the coffin, allowing the others to lay a red and dark blue blanket under it. Then the four men lifted the four corners of the blanket with the coffin and lowered it into the grave. I saw a triangular piece of yellow in the blanket as it was lowered, sagging with the weight of the coffin. The mother never flinched.

With my head above the two rows of people in front of me, I saw two boys emerge out of the circle with two shovels each, and the four men began shoveling the pile of dirt on top of the coffin. You could hear the sickening sound of dirt hitting wood. No one else moved, but I could hear crying. The monk in orange reappeared. He said some prayers and many in the crowd joined in. The mother did not. Then, in response to words from the monk, the crowd began to disperse. I looked for the woman in white silk, but she was gone.

While reversing direction on the path, the Vietnamese nurse walked along side of me, taking two skipped steps to my one. Miss Tam explained, "In Vietnam, family cum back after tree months an sit. Only family. Monk put cotton over head an ring bell an dey pray. Dey want bring spirit back. After dey burn paper house an odder paper things, den spirit come back from odder world." I thought it was no more ridiculous than the malarkey that I was brought up on.

We reached the main road and before we parted, the nurse said, "I go home now. Very sad. Girl die from too much smoke from bomb from sky." Nodding my head, I felt intense shame.

I hitched a ride in an American deuce and a half to get back to my base. Standing in the open back of the truck looking at glimpses of the wide Mekong River through thick vegetation—glimmers of water and flat boats and shacks—I didn't even know the cause of the respiratory distress that killed Lan. Our bomb. And I realized that while Lan was wrapped in the colors of the South Vietnamese flag, her coffin lay on top of the red and dark blue blanket, and the triangular yellow was part of a star: the colors of the Viet Cong flag.

The Monsoon's blinding rain came without warning as if the sky just opened up and dumped all that it had stored up. I took my cap off and lifted my arms heavenward, allowing the water to run down my body.

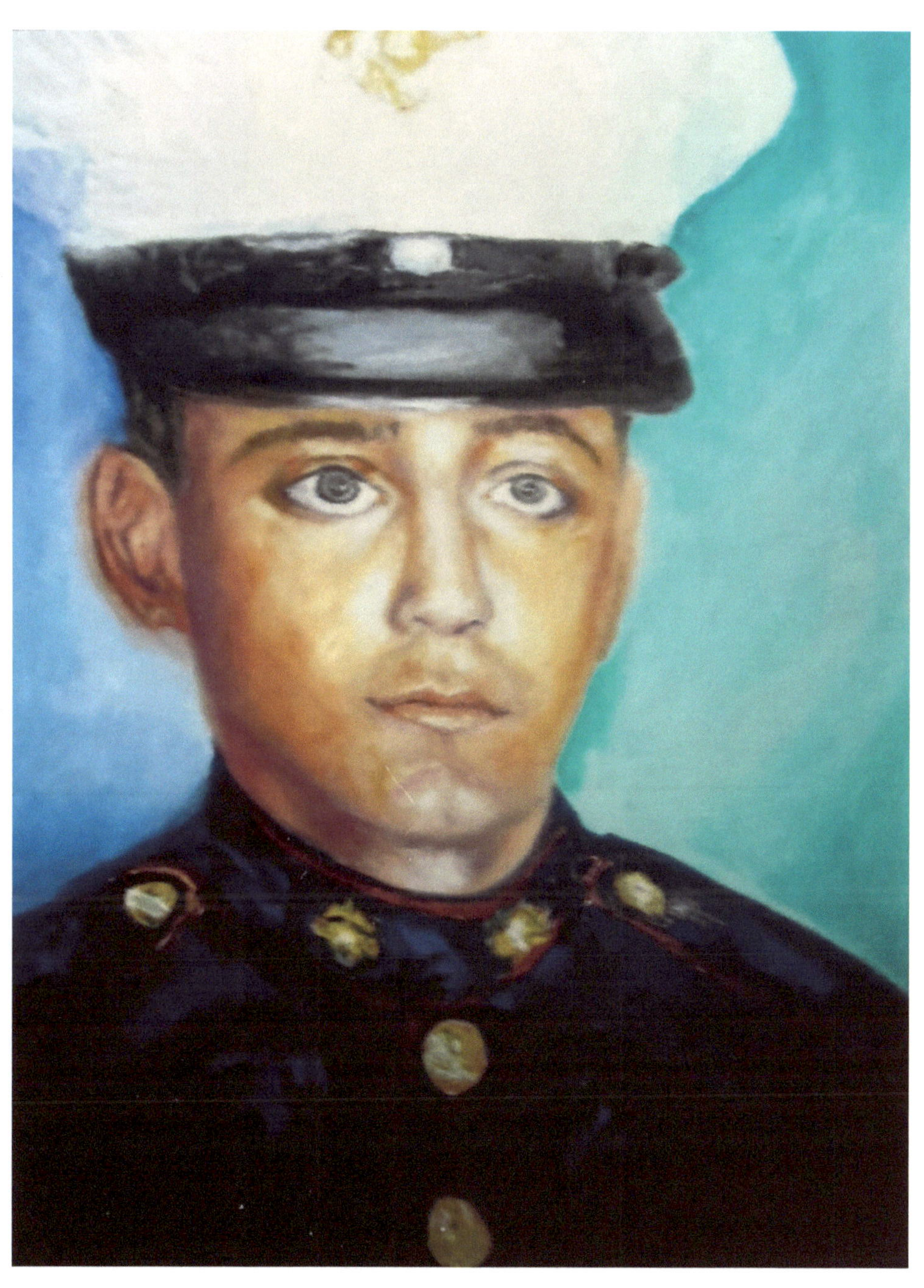

James Carloni, Age 19
Vietnam, KIA
Private Collection

An Everyday Incident that Chips Away at the Spirit

The locker room reeked of sweat and was filled with loud, irritating rap music. Wedged in-between rows of tall, dark green metal lockers, a familiar feeling of claustrophobia set in as I rushed through the uncomfortable routine of undressing as if all eyes were on me. Pulling up my white gym shorts, I looked to my left and nodded to a tall black kid with a reddish-brown Afro; he was shirtless, muscular, probably in his late teens. While maintaining a serious face, he answered with a barely perceptible lowering of his chin. After putting a padlock on my locker, I walked into the gym but came to a halt upon seeing the treadmills; I forgot my I-Pod.

When I opened my combination lock on the tall metal door, it felt like a hand was squeezing my throat and my heart was pounding against my ribcage. Everything was gone, including my wallet with credit cards and over $200.

I asked the black kid, "Did you see anyone take anything out of this locker?"

Turning his head and looking at me with a scowl, he answered in a deep voice, "I don't know nothing about your locker."

He had an unbuttoned black dress shirt on that dropped to his thighs, and I watched him bend over and put his shorts into a huge white gym bag in slow motion. While the kid's face was above the gym bag, his left eye was still on me.

"I wasn't gone more than a minute. Someone took all my stuff! You didn't see anyone near my locker?"

The black kid stood up and turned his body to face me. "I told you I don't know nothing about your locker."

With a quiver in my voice, I answered, "O.K. I just wondered if you saw something."

Why the anger? Was that a sign of guilt? Or was he annoyed about what looked and sounded to him as being unjustly accused.

Did I have the look of suspicion when I asked the question? I was upset. I would have had the same look and tone if the kid was white.

I ran down the long stairway, teeth clinched and breathing rapidly, wondering how was it possible the kid didn't see anything when he was less than 10 feet away. And his white gym bag was huge.

I informed a young woman at the front desk what had happened and asked her to call the police.

While leaning my back against the front counter, I watched the same black kid wearing a light grey hoodie over his head descend the steps. He looked to his left at me like he smelled something bad. I jerked my head forward, but I kept my eyes on him through the large front glass window as he entered a car waiting in the dark with hazard lights blinking. Snow was gently falling but with the inside car light on, I saw that the driver looked like an older black guy.

I felt fear as the car remained parked in front flashing bursts of light into the night and with both heads turned toward me.

***

Two young, tall police officers arrived, dressed in navy blue shirts and ties with silver badges on their left breast. I informed them about the robbery. The three of us went up the stairs; I hesitated on a step half way up but decided to delay saying anything about the black guys parked in front.

On the way to the locker room, I thought that by hanging around, it was unlikely that the kid took my stuff, but it occurred to me that he might want to kick my ass.

With the cops hovering over me, I pointed to the empty locker and exclaimed, "I don't know why they bothered to put the lock back on. Why would anyone take my underwear?"

One of the officer's looked inside the next locker to my right and asked, "This locker has clothes in it. Is this your stuff?"

I looked into the other locker. It was my stuff. I put my clothes in that locker and while momentarily distracted by the black kid's annoyance at me nodding at him, put the padlock on the next empty locker. I was mortified.

***

I skipped my shower and while packing my bag, I was afraid the two black guys might be still waiting for me. It was not likely that a son and father would kick the shit out of me. But I thought it was probable that the father would angerly confront me about falsely accusing his son. Why else would they wait? But I didn't accuse anyone.

Upset that I didn't walk out with the cops, I quickly descended the stairs, but I paused at the door to see if the kid and his father were still waiting for me. Between the blinding white light I was standing under and the blowing, swirling snow outside, I couldn't see inside the parked car, but the lights were still blinking. I took a deep breath and stepped out into the frigid night air, watching cold clouds of my hyperventilating breath rise and dissipate. I stood and scanned the parking lot, acting ever so nonchalantly, avoiding the blinking car to my left. There were only a few scattered cars and not a soul around; it was eerily silent. I walked briskly to my car, immediately locked myself in, and called my wife, initiating an unnecessary conversation that lasted at least 10 minutes. Driving past the gym entrance on my way out of the parking lot, I casually looked to my left. There was still a car in front of the gym with flashing lights, but it was a different car with two guys in the front seat. Two white guys.

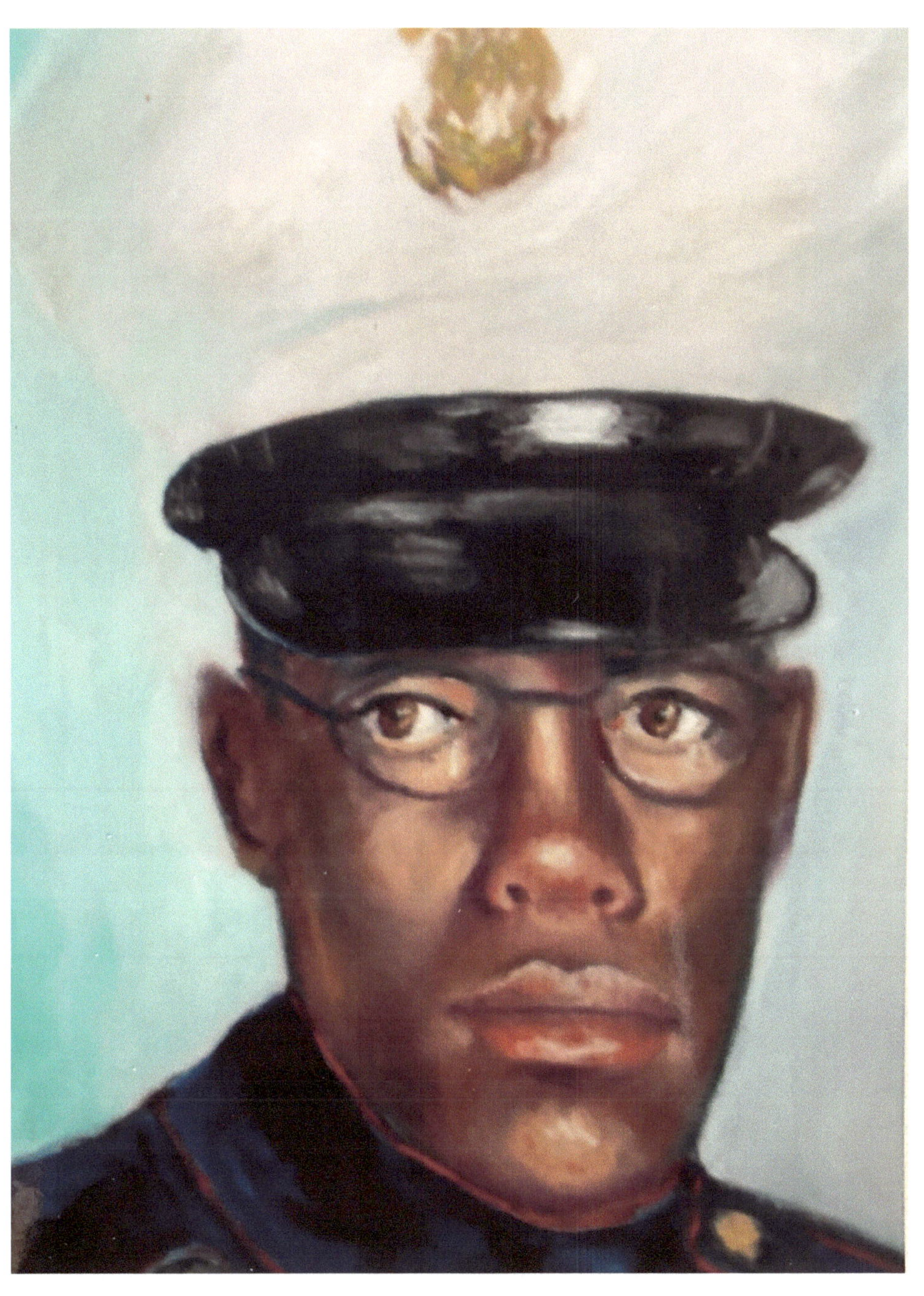

Joe
Vietnam
NYC VA Regional Office Museum

Why Was Jesus Laughing?

Jesus, laughing so hard his head was falling backward with his face heavenward and flashing upper teeth made whiter by his brown skin. I rarely looked up to see my mother's painting of him; it was round in shape and its size was no bigger than a common plate, mimicking the clock that ticked next to it. The oil on canvas image hung in the kitchen for years rarely provoking a word during thousands of meals in my adolescence, our family of four in binding silence imposed by my father.

Why was Jesus laughing? He would have undoubtedly found the pairing of a tiny, fiery artist from the toe of Italy's boot with a big brooding Irishman hilarious. But I had seen many images of Jesus in my mother's art books; he was either hanging on the cross or dead in his mother's arms. I never saw him laughing.

Seated in the kitchen with eyes downcast, our father gave his blessing for his first born to volunteered at the height of the Vietnam war. His consecration of the patriotic act was based on the belief that by being a good soldier of Christ Jesus, one can attain salvation through suffering.

My older brother came home from Vietnam on the heels of the Battle of Khe Sanh. Patrick, sitting under the painting of Jesus, frequently nodded out during supper. We knew he was spiritually hollow and emotionally numb. We feared he would die. Yet we sat around the table like Picasso's La Famille de Saltimbanques, looking in different directions at nothing in particular.

***

The houses in South Buffalo were so close to one another that you could barely fit a car between them, two story wooden structures with porches and comfortable gliders, and people shouting pleasantries to their neighbors over the din of their kids playing in the yards and street. The community was predominately blue-collar Irish Catholic, filled with children sharing bedrooms with bunkbeds. There were steelworkers, mechanics, firemen, and cops with a few politicians in the mix. Nearly every brood was served daily rations of cold, harsh discipline and mass on Sunday. Those old enough or with a fake ID flocked to the corner bars seeking warmth and relief. The draft was on the horizon with Vietnam looming, but coming home covered in steel mill coal dust, I couldn't think past the night in front of me.

On an ugly Friday night in late November, I staggered back home after last call, cursing into an icy wind slapping my face. Since the kitchen light was on, I knew my father would be sitting at the table. I wasn't afraid of him anymore. Not with a load on anyway.

I opened the side door and saw my parents sitting at the kitchen table. My mother was quietly sobbing on her forearms, her long grey hair spilled over half the table. My father looked at me with vacuous eyes.

I mumbled, "What's going on?"

My father responded, "Your brother is dead."

"What?"

My father was a World War II Marine who never spoke of the horrors of Iwo Jima and Okinawa except in bursts when drunk or in nightmares. Cut out of a block of granite with a grey crew-cut, huge hands, and grim face, he said in a low monotone voice, "A Buffalo police officer just left. He said Patrick died of a heroin overdose three hours ago."

It took a few seconds to process what my father said. I became very light-headed and dizzy. With hands on the table, I steadied myself and asked my father, "Couldn't there be a mistake?"

My mother raised her head and turned to my father with a pleading expression, searching for some sign of hope in her husband's face.

Crushing an empty beer can with his massive right hand, my father said with brutal finality, "The police officer brought Patrick's personal things: his watch, wallet, and keys."

My mother and I stared at each other in disbelief, choking on our grief.

My father asked me to go up to Patrick's bedroom closet to get a toolbox. I did what I was told. The rectangular silver box was on the floor, only partially covered with clothes. I used my right foot to slide the clothes off the metal box and picked it up. Walking downstairs and returning to the kitchen, I thought of how different he was away from the tomb where we broke bread. My brother was affable like our mother with a quick wit and talked with great passion using his hands. But he returned a stranger.

I placed the silver metal box in the middle of the table. There was a thick padlock guarding its contents.

As if in a trance, my father walked into the garage and came back with a hammer and screwdriver. He hit the screwdriver on the lock with the hammer multiple times. We shook with each blow. The lock finally broke into pieces, flying in different directions, one hitting my leg before landing on the floor. When he opened the steel box, we saw the contents: a stack of baseball cards held together by a rubber band with Patrick's prized Mickey Mantle on top, three syringes, a rubber hose, and four small cellophane bags with white powder.

In a barely audible voice, my father asked me, "Did you know anything about this?"

I avoided my father's eyes while replying, "No. I would have said something if I knew Patrick's was using that stuff. I mean marijuana wouldn't surprise me but heroin? I can't believe he was shooting heroin."

My father looked at me and asked through gritted teeth, "Have you ever used drugs?"

I answered, "No Dad. No way. I don't do drugs."

"The officer who just left said your brother was found in drug house near Filmore and Broadway, the most crime infested part of the city. I don't understand how—. Do you know anything about this place?"

"No. I would never go anywhere near there."

When I looked up, I saw Jesus laughing, his frizzy dark hair hung down to his mid-back, his beard of the same color and texture covering an elevated chin. I remembered my father once complaining bitterly about the dark skin and the laughing to my mother, growling, "He was not that dark and had nothing to laugh about!"

Standing toe to toe with him, my mother looked up at her husband and said, "He was a middle eastern Jew 2,000 years ago. And he sees plenty to laugh about."

My father preferred a Jesus back on the cross, his white elongated, twisted body suffering.

I looked at Jesus laughing. He knew of his impending torture and death, but he must have anticipated his resurrection. Maybe that's why his laugh was raucous. Or despite witnessing all of his miracles and listening to all his teaching firsthand, some of his disciples would betray and abandon him. Was that the joke?

My parents sat frozen in shock. No one was trying to comfort anyone. It was as if Patrick lay dead on that table, surrounded by mourners unable to fully comprehend what had happened. Just weeks earlier, he had survived a ferocious enemy attack of many weeks' duration. My mother's forehead sunk back into her forearms, her long grey hair still spilled out before her, weeping, repeating her dead son's name. My father looked at her with drooping eyes, swallowing.

My old man knew about the toolbox. If he had suspicions, why didn't he make Patrick open it? I also knew about the box. I suspected it contained drugs, but I never asked my brother about it.

Listening to my mother weeping, I wanted to shout: "You leave no stone unturned in this house. Why didn't you speak up?"

Patrick left the silver box partially visible as a cry for help we chose to ignore. We let our flesh and blood drown in front of our eyes.

***

After making a phone call, my father asked me to drive him to the morgue. We walked into a bright white room and saw a gurney with a white sheet pulled over a shape of a supine body. After exchanging names, a very tall, thin, middle-aged man wearing a long white hospital coat pulled the white sheet up and across the body, revealing a head, bare chest, and shoulders. The face had a pale-bluish hue, but it was Patrick with his long, curly brown hair and wispy go-tee. I had to hold my father up. I guided him into a chair. He gasped—I saw deep crevasses in-between his eyebrows—but he snapped back to stoicism.

I felt no emotion at seeing my brother's cold, lifeless face. I grew up watching my father stuff all his emotions except rage. And I resented my brother; a hero in life and martyr in death. But Patrick never found what he was looking for from my father, an impassive man who had also seen unspeakable horrors. Our father had nothing to give. And after the death of his favored son, he stopped praying.

***

The following spring, I stood in the driveway watching my mother paint. With a stretched canvas on wooden easel in front of our home, a pregnant woman pushing a baby buggy paused to marvel at flowers bursting off the canvas in shades of red, yellow, purple, and orange. As the sun set, I helped my mother drag her painting and materials into our basement. She labored late into the night, as if it were penance, only to leave her unfinished work to languish in our dank cellar.

A robust man of 6 feet, my father seemed to shrink. I watched him sink in his black leather chair looking at the television, but I could tell he was not processing anything. He would fall asleep in that chair, night after night. I stood over him once and looked down upon the back of his shock of white hair. I felt pity, but it was fleeting.

As summer drew near, the painting of Jesus laughing disappeared. My mother believed my father had thrown it out. He denied it, but she didn't believe him. I let them argue. I took the painting. I couldn't walk into the kitchen without looking up at Jesus and feeling rage. Salvation? It's a lie. That's why Jesus was laughing.

The following evening, while sitting at the kitchen table with my spent parents, I confessed, "I put the painting next to the slab of cement that marks what's left of my brother's dead body."

***

In front of our home on Bloomfield Street, every spring, there was a long row of Peonies. There were puffy blossoms with colors of white, pink, rose, and red. But Buffalo has no spring; the flowers lose their color and die so soon.

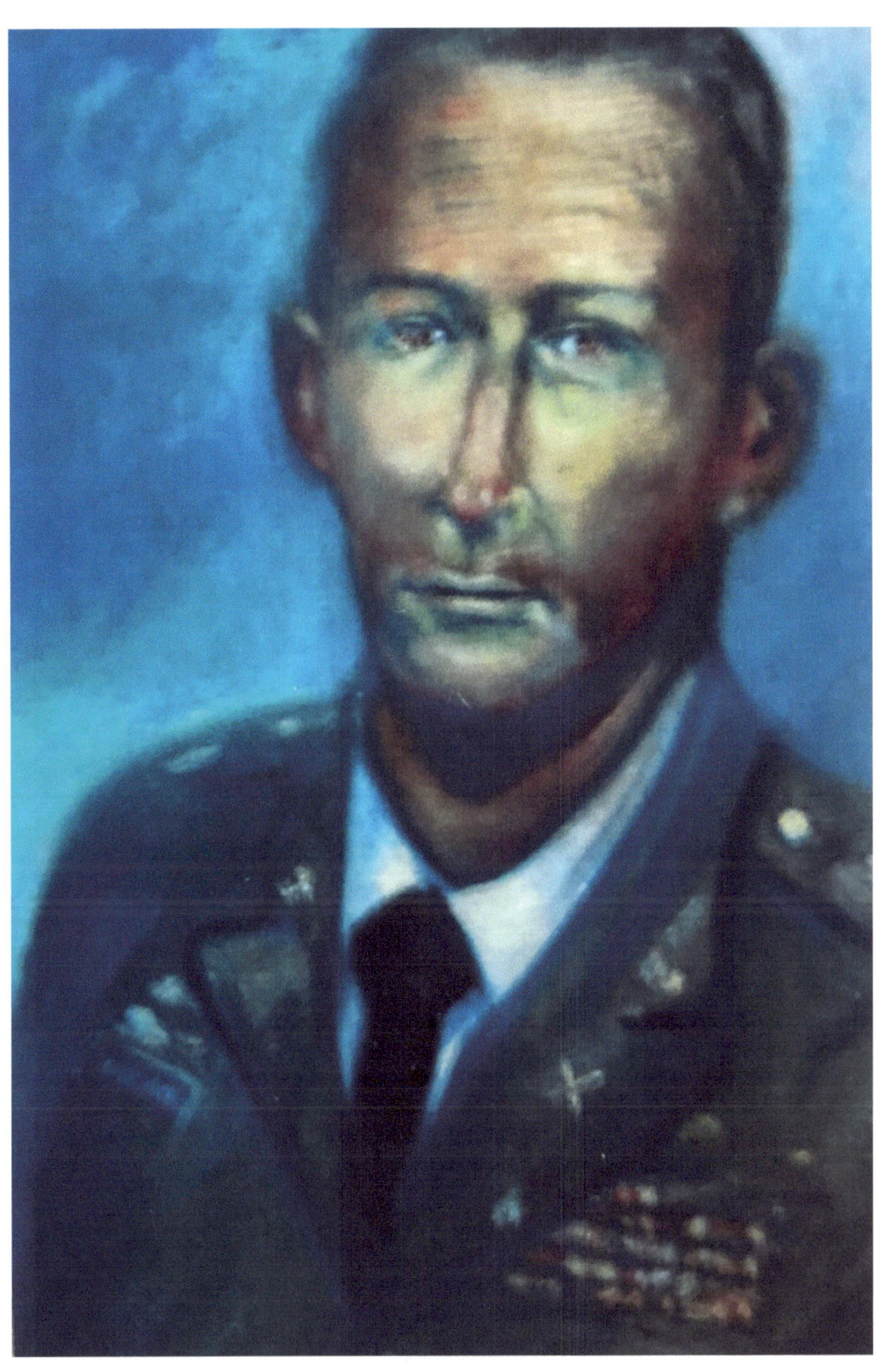

Mike Duggan
Vietnam
Private Collection

Ciao Jackie Jocko

My partner, Joe Paolucci rushed into my dressing room yelling, "Jackie, Jackie, you're not going to believe this! Follow me to Sinatra's dressing room. Get your clothes back on. Come on."

I shouted, "Sinatra's dressing room? What the hell are you talking about? This is gotta be some kind of a joke."

"No joke Jackie. But he ain't gonna wait all night."

Tall, dark and with a full head of thick, dyed black hair and a hairline just above his eyebrows, Joe had a hunchback that still left him 6 inches taller than me. He had a long Roman nose and a face chiseled out of Michelangelo's marble quarry. My partner had no capacity to lie or laugh.

Struck with horror at my nude, egg-shaped image in a full-length mirror, I slowly put my oversized tux back on, slicked my thin, black toupee to the right, and walked with trepidation down a narrow hall toward a blinding light. Joe and I had been opening for Sinatra at The Sands for the past 4 nights, with one more to go, and the most I got from the Chairman was a nod and a smile. He said, "Hey there" once, but he was looking past me. Sinatra was always followed by his entourage and surrounded by admirers. I didn't think anyone outside of his inner circle could get close to his dressing room, let alone in it. I suspected a cruel hoax.

As I approached Joe, he was uncharacteristically rubbing his palms, wild-eyed, waiting at Sinatra's door. Twenty-five years I lived with this guy; his normal demeanor was barely a notch above corpse. Rocking back and forth on the balls of his feet, he cried, "Go on in Jackie. You're not going to believe this."

I looked up at Joe and said, "Gimmie some of whatever you're smoking."

The door was open and I followed Joe's hunchback in like a running back. The room was huge with many mirrors; chairs and tables; a large white leather couch; and what looked like part of a brass bed behind curtains. As my head slowly turned, I saw a solid oak bar, the color of sand. There must have been over 100 bottles of booze on shelves behind the bar and many photos of Frank with different people, most gorgeous, all famous.

The dozen or more chattering people were a blur; my eyes focused on Sinatra holding up a rock glass with caramel colored liquid over ice. Looking at me squarely in the eyes, he bellowed, "Happy birthday John Giaccio! Fifty is the big one mi paisano!" He flashed his beautiful white teeth, but it was his azure blue eyes that were mesmerizing. It was the first time I was able to look into his eyes.

I looked at a round glass table next to Frank; a huge rectangular cake sat in the middle, with Happy Birthday Jackie written in white icing on a thick layer of chocolate frosting. I could smell the chocolate. Someone, probably Joe, arranged for the cake to be covered in dozens of flaming candles. Still buzzing, all eyes were on me. In Sinatra's room! Me?

Frank put his drink on a dresser, extended his arms out, gave me a bear hug, and softly said in my right ear, "John Giaccio, play buon cumpleanno and I'll sing it for you."

I wondered how Sinatra knew my real name. It had been at least 20 years since anyone addressed me by anything other than my stage name, Jackie Jocko. Joe must have set this up, but how did he get Sinatra to go along? By this time in the evening, Frank would probably be behind that curtain with some dame.

The crowd behind Sinatra parted as if on cue, revealing a baby grand piano. I admired the ebony that shined and its brilliant white keys. It was the most beautiful piano I had ever seen.

With legs of rubber, I don't know how I managed to walk to the piano. With my left hand on the piano to steady myself, I felt disbelief mixed with rapture while floating as if in a dream. I briefly recalled the morphine-induced euphoria I experienced following back surgery. This was better. But in the far recesses of my mind, I was waiting for the other shoe to drop.

I sat down at the piano and managed a meek, "Sure Frank. You bet."

I began playing something I had not played for more than 30 years. Frank, standing to my left but within my peripheral vision, looked around the room as he sang the birthday song, but his eyes kept returning to me.

When we finished the song and acknowledged the applause, tears were streaming down my face upon seeing Frank Sinatra and his people saluting me. The clapping continued while I stood up and bowed several times. After the applause finally stopped, Frank walked over and gave me another hug, while whispering in my right ear, "Happy birthday my gumba." Good friend? Then he kissed me on the right cheek. The whole scene was surreal. But part of me felt like I deserved the respect. Thirty years on the circuit, always the introducing act; that I had finally arrived was no fluke. Joe and I had paid our dues.

I looked for Joe, but I couldn't find him in the crowd.

As much as I adored the attention, I was vividly sensing another person in the room. As my eyes scanned the gathering, I saw a couple dressed exactly alike, with skin tight green and yellow plaid suits, and red corn-rolled wigs atop faces with gleaming white and red paint. A boy, no more than 12, with straight brown hair, squeezed through the clowns. His bangs dropped to his eyebrows, and he had a sweet angelic face, like one Raphael's cherubs. The boy was dressed in a white suit and white cap, standing alone and somber. I remembered my first communion.

Where did I know this boy? Haunting lyrics meandered through my brain:
"We looked at each other in the same way then
But I can't remember where or when …"

Suddenly it came to me: Vicente Calvizzano from my old Fillmore and East Delevan neighborhood. But no; that was decades ago.

While shaking hands with well-wishers, my mind traveled back to my 8th birthday party and Vicente was there. He was four years older than me. Dressed in a dark brown suit that was too small for him, with his trousers above his ankles, Vicente had just arrived from Italy. His parents brought him from San Fele, a town in the province of Potenza, the same town that my parents came from. Half of my Buffalo neighborhood was from that town in central Italy; they traveled on overcrowded buses to Naples and a huge ship brought them to the American dream. Buffalo was no shining city on a hill, but there was work. Friends, relatives, and neighbors, voyaging to settle with familiar faces and tongue.

Why was I having such thoughts with Sinatra in the room?

I suddenly had a nostalgic remembrance upon the realization that I had never felt as happy as the day of my 8th birthday party. My mother was there, short and stout, wearing a simple black dress that went to her ankles, with dark bags under her eyes and unkempt, thinning grey hair. Her sitting in a chair revealed rumpled stockings above high top, collapsing black shoes; you couldn't dress more unattractive if you tried, but we were poor and she was beautiful in my eyes. My father died several years earlier, but my mama stayed in that faded black dress until her death 20 years later. I have no image of my father other than his screaming in Italian and beating my rear-end with his heavily callused hand. I can't visualize his face nor the home I grew up in other than an old piano in the middle of the living room, with wobbly legs and many scars.

I could see Vicente's mother, also perpetually wearing a black dress, yelling from inside a screened door in Italian, "Vicente, Vieni a cena. Com e mangiare." She was calling him to supper in her sing song voice. From wherever he was, Vicente always came running home in his threadbare knickers and brown shoes full of holes.

There were many old women at my 8th birthday party, almost all dressed in simple widow black over their small round figures, their husband's war-torn bodies buried in Italy, France, or some South Pacific island.

Vicente took piano lessons from the same lady who taught me, a tiny grey-haired woman with wrinkles in her gaunt face, granny glasses on the tip of her large nose, and long delicate fingers. But he was far behind me because I started at age 3. Our mothers worked, scrimped, and saved to pay for those lessons.

Vicente was my hero. I was small for my age and was bullied on occasion. Some fat kid was on top of me in the school playground, ready to give another blow to the head when Vicente came to my rescue. He picked the fat kid up by the collar, turned him around by the shoulders, and punched him in the gut. The bully ran away, squealing like a pig. He never bothered me again.

When Vicente turned 18, he left our neighborhood to fight the Nazis. We were embarrassed by Mussolini, but proud of our fathers and boys. I remember the day Vicente went to the train that took him away, slim and handsome in his dark three-piece brown suit; white shirt; and a short, wide dark brown tie. His hair was black and wet, combed straight back, and he had skin of ivory without a blemish. He gave me a wink. I never saw him again. He was killed on the beach of Salerno.

I was standing outside of a circle that surrounded Sinatra, but was distracted by scenes of Napoli, where I walked through neighborhoods with clothes hung out to dry on fire escapes and streets full of waddling women wearing scarfs and children running amok. Many adults were yelling with arms flailing about; they sounded like arguments, but I knew most were not. I saw boys in short pants kicking a soccer ball in the street. I remember leaving San Fele on a rickety bus going up and down dirt roads on hills. Looking out the window, I saw old men wearing black caps in a park playing bocce. I was choking on a ball of fear in my throat; I was never in the old country.

I woke up. I looked at my hands and saw many ugly brown spots, prominent veins zigzagging on top of wrinkled skin, fingers grotesquely twisted, and every small joint swollen. My heart sunk. When I stepped out of that dream, I had aged 40 years. From a robust middle-aged man with a strong, melodious voice to a bent over, decrepit dotard, singing weak, cracked sounds that are often no more than a whisper. Someone recently told me, probably after looking at my hands, that Renoir, at 90, was able to keep painting with paint brushes taped to his hands. Good for him. But my fingers must hit the keys with dexterity, as they have done for the past 84 years. I don't know how I do it five nights a week. I say to myself in the mirror on a daily basis, "Quit while you are not too far behind Jocko."

I grimaced from pain in my back and hips as I swung my legs out of my bed. I had to catch my breath before using my hands to lift myself up and stand. Joe is gone. I moan and curse as loud as I want now, but I don't like being alone. I staggered to the bathroom to be met by drooping jowls and large wrinkled, bluish sacks under my eyes. Holding my shriveled-up penis, the urine took its usual long time and it hurt. Everything hurt. I went back to bed and tried to slip into that dream with Sinatra and Vicente, but like a bubble, it burst without leaving a trace. I tossed and turned my old flesh covering aching and brittle bones. My ankles and feet were filled with fluid and ice cold. My heart doesn't pump anymore; it quivers.

The taxi takes me down many dark streets to sit at the large black baby grand piano at EB Green's lounge, my little oasis. I leave exhausted, and the cab takes me back through the gutter to a cold, empty house. The only thing left is my music If I could choose a perpetual dream in death, would it be in Sinatra's dressing room with Frank, Joe, and a ghost? No. It would be at my 8th birthday party with flesh and blood: Vicente in his white suit and me, sweet birds of youth, and my tired mother in widow black.

I forget almost all of my dreams but not that one. Sitting at the kitchen table in my black robe and red fluffy slippers, Humpty Dumpty with a cup of black coffee, I tried to analyze the dream. Some who know such things say dreams are projections of parts of the self that have been suppressed. Did Sinatra represent an aspect of me? Did the boy Vicente? Others say inanimate objects can represent aspects of the dreamer too. The boy, Frank, and the piano—it isn't hard to figure out.

Later that day, I suited up in my tux and toupee. William Anthony Hooper, the owner of the restaurant, insists on this. I have shrunk in old age and look like a jockey, swimming in a monkey suit. I am a marionette and Signor Hooper pulls the strings, but I am compelled to entertain. That's all I got.

Arriving at E.B. Green's, I dragged my tired old body into the cocktail lounge. My organs are barely functioning; I think some have shut down. A heavy sadness enveloped me as I shuffled in. But not when my fingers hit the shimmering white keys of the shiny black piano; I sometimes feel like

I did in the dream. In a zone aglow, I make music and people respond with their lips and eyes. For a dozen hour a week, before the pain returns, I am enveloped in bliss.

I scooped up the tips in a white porcelain dish on the piano and shuffled out, too bushed to say my usual personal good-byes. I prayed to Jesus and the Blessed Virgin: please take me. I desperately want to go back to that dream and stay there. I want Joe, Vicente, and a magnificent polished black piano in the room. And will my mother be there if I wish and pray it so? I don't give a damn about Sinatra.

I can't go back. But my friends come every night: Howie and Fran Goldberg pawing each other; Joey G with his brass horn on his knee; a cute, petite blonde named Suzie; Starburst with her big fake tits; and Louie Pep with his perpetual heebie-jeebies. When their faces tell me to continue playing, I forget about my deformed fingers, twisted spine, and crushing despair.

Don't ever put me out to pasture in some home for the half dead, slumped in a wheelchair or sitting on a bedpan. Give me some powerful drug so that I will drift into a permanent sleep. Ciao Jacki Jocko.

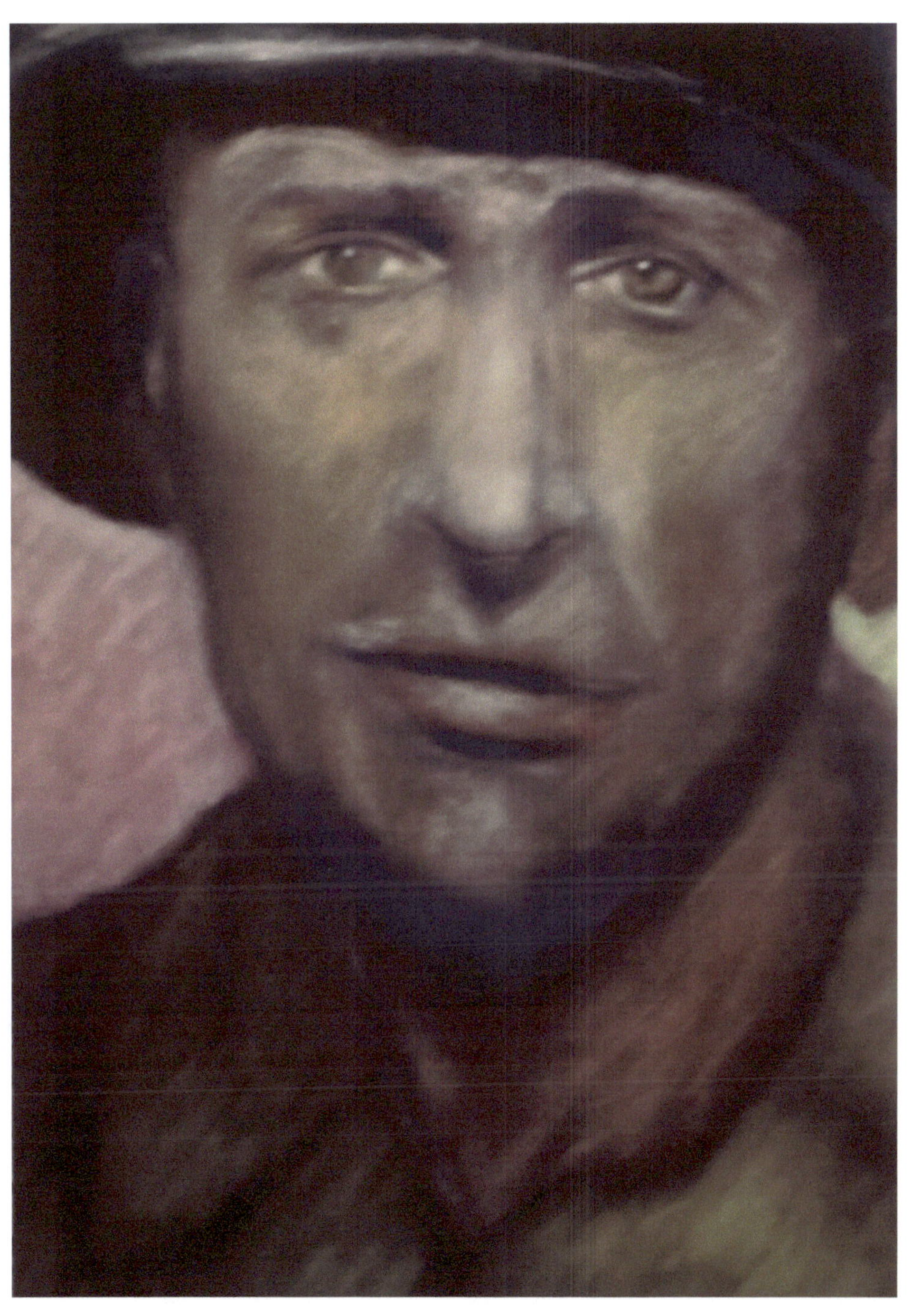

David, Age 28
WWII, Battle of the Bulge , KIA
Private Collection

Not Asking for Help

I had no idea how to use an I-Phone. The technology was changing so fast that it ran past me, and I had no desire to try and catch up. I longed for a simpler time when there was just an on and off switch. Being an old gringo who traveled frequently from New York City to various parts of Latin America, it didn't matter where I hung my hat; with respect to electronics, it was always no country for old men.

But my wife persisted and after seeing people tapping such phones everywhere—even old men—I threw in the towel. It was slim and sleek and I particularly liked my new ability of looking up names of people, places, and things I kept forgetting. And in the weeks preceding our vacation in Mexico, I finally got the hang of taking photos and short films and sending them to friends with a text. I fancied myself quite clever in linking colorful words with vivid images.

The sun brought welcome warmth to my face, but it was still chilly at noon on a January day in San Miguel de Allende, located more than a mile up in the heart of Mexico. I looked at Lola 20 yards ahead on the narrow cobblestone street winding down and curving to the left. Dressed in white slacks and a black sweater with big Gucci sunglasses, she was crouching down and fingering through some trinkets while speaking Spanish to an old woman in a crimson red serape, sitting on a cement door step next to her colorful wares spread over a black blanket.

I yelled, "I'll catch up. I want to take a photo."

An intricately carved exotic bird—graceful with its long-curved neck and thin legs—was on a tall rectangular door covered with peeling turquois paint that stopped me in my tracks. Ahh! My first stunning photo and we just stepped out of our hotel. The yellow ocher surrounding the door was perfect foil for the turquois. You have to have a good eye for great pictures and I had it.

But when I took my I-phone out of a black leather pouch strapped to my waist and tried to take a photo, instead of seeing the object of interest,

I saw black. I tapped the icon to turn the camera eye on me and there I was, but a tap to flip back to the turquois door revealed a black screen. I went to settings and began a series of touching every possibility, adding and withdrawing apps. Nada.

I walked briskly down the winding cobblestone street, following Lola's auburn hair falling down over her shoulders, upset as I saw additional photo opportunities. I stopped a few steps from the lady with the knick-knacks. She was sitting next to her black blanket covered with a wide array of carved wooden animals painted in reds, blues, and yellows. The tiny brown-skinned lady, squinting into the sun while looking up at me, had sunken black eyes with deep crevices and spider wrinkles covering most of her face. Seeing the photo opportunity, I gave her 50 pesos for a tiny cerulean blue wooden donkey. After stuffing the donkey in my back pocket, I tried shutting the phone off, turning it on, and tapping through all of the possible combinations again. Still black.

I found my wife sitting comfortably in an outdoor café on a folding wooden chair, hands clasped on a round wooden table covered by a fuchsia table cloth, surveying the scenery. There were yellow and red flowers in the middle of the table; the iconic Virgin of Guadalupe was on both sides of the white porcelain vase.

"Listen Louis, I'm starving so I'm ordering something. What took you so long?"

Holding my phone in front of Lola's face, I explained my dilemma and added, "I went to settings and turned on and off every stinking thing in there. I connected this with that in every possible combination to no avail."

My wife's big eyes lifted over the menu she was reading, exasperated at my whining. She asked, "Why don't you ask the waiter? He's a young guy and can probably figure it out."

Shaking my head, I replied, "There's absolutely nothing I haven't tried. I need to go to an Apple Store but lots of luck finding one here. "Besides, I don't want anyone pulling apart my new phone. I don't get it. How can it be O.K. on one side and not on the other? I'm in this beautiful town and I can't take one lousy photo."

"But you don't know what you're doing with this kind of stuff. It could be something simple."

"Simple? I've been fooling around with this stupid thing for a half hour. There's nothing simple about it."

A short, thin young man appeared with a tuft of black hair stiffened into a point, wearing an open-collared white shirt. Lola put her menu down and asked the waiter, "How are the fish tacos?"

The waiter smiled broadly and answered, "Excellent señora! They are the best in San Miguel."

"Are they big? I see an order has 3."

"No señora. They are not too big. An order of 3 is perfect."

"All right. One order of fish tacos with everything and a glass of white wine. The Chablis please."

As I shifted in my wooden chair trying to find a comfortable position, the old lady's wooden donkey was digging into my right buttock. I snapped at the waiter, "A glass of Pinot noir. No. Make that a bottle of Pinot."

"Si señor."

I pulled the donkey out of my ass and slapped it on the table. My wife frowned and said, "Boy are you in one foul mood. Here we are in this lovely town on a beautiful day on a vacation we desperately need and all you do is complain. We might as well go back to—"

"I know. I'm sorry. It's this goddamn phone."

"Louis, put the phone away. Order some food. Relax. Most people waste so much time with their camera that they miss the whole experience."

"I suppose that's true. But I'd at least like to have a record of some of it."

The waiter came back with the wine. I held the bottle and as I slowly poured the wine into my glass, I was distracted by a tiny old lady with a high stack of wide-brimmed hats on her head and knocked my glass over, spilling the wine.

"Son of a fucking bitch!"

"Louis please. There are people all around us. It's not a big deal. Calm down."

I looked around at the surrounding outdoor tables. All eyes were on me. One old gringo with a knapsack and a grey pony tail from what hair remained on the back of his head looked at me with pursed lip contempt. I glared while noticing he had a knapsack like a school child and wore Birkenstock shoes. I slowly and silently articulated with a wide-open mouth, "Fuck-you asshole."

The lady selling the sombreros stepped a few paces back. Gazing at her colorful indigenous dress with blue and red flowers and that leaning tower of hats, I seethed, "Another great picture missed."

However, after my second full glass of wine on an empty stomach, I put things in their proper perspective, realizing that this was not even a half of our first day. And I conceded Lola was right regarding my urgency of taking photos; our visit must be about seeing and feeling each exhilarating experience.

As I watched my wife devour her fish tacos, I was amazed at how she could eat them loaded up with white fish, light green avocado, strings of onions, and coleslaw bulging out of the edges of the yellow corn tortilla without dropping a speck. It was all in her hands and leaning forward over the plate. When I eat tacos, the contents end up all over my shirt. Of course, having grown up in Mexico, she had home field advantage.

Feeling mellow, I marveled at how Lola hadn't aged much in the last 20 years: bronze complexion without a wrinkle, that long chestnut hair draped over her shoulders, big Latin eyes with increased space between the eyebrow and very long eyelash and a crease through the middle of that space, and natural full lips. (At 6 foot, 3 inches, I'm a foot taller than my wife, and my white hair and beard makes me look 10 years older, but that doesn't bother either of us. It's my mouth that gets me into trouble.)

When the young waiter reappeared asking if we needed anything, my wife asked in Spanish, "Can you help my husband with his phone?"

Before the waiter could answer, I said through a smirk, "No. Thank-you but no. I'll figure this out."

Looking perplexed, the waiter withdrew.

Lola and I walked holding hands. Feeling the wine, I found San Miguel an enchanting city of stone: the sidewalks are light grey; the streets are filled with cobblestones of the same color, and the colonial buildings of two and three stories—there's nothing taller except for the towers of old ornate churches—consist of smooth stone painted Indian red and different hues of yellow but subdued, which is in stark contrast to the ever-present flock of revelers in the streets.

Looking at street after immaculate street without seeing a garbage can, I wrapped a piece of tasteless gum in its wrapper and stuck it in my pocket. Walking slowly, exploring shops, we saw many arches surrounding garden patios inside, Hacienda-style. There were cacti of many sizes and shapes in some of the gardens; more than a few looked like excited people with arms up or bodies bent forward and backward. One reminded me of an exclamation point with its fat, rounded top and tapered bottom.

That first evening, we sat on the north edge of the Jardin, a beautiful square park in the middle of the city, full of trees and people of all ages, facing the front of an unusual cathedral for Mexico: a huge Gothic-like structure, baroque with soaring pale pink spires. It looked like something out of 17th century Western Europe. A flock of large white birds shot out of the spires upon the sound of loud bells.

As we were licking ice cream cones trying to beat the melt, an incredible scene began to unfold. Mariachis atop a dozen black horses high stepped and stopped in two perfect horizontal lines about 50 yards in front of the massive church, and we had ring-side seats of approximately the same distance from the other side of that spectacular vision. The men wore familiar large white conical sombreros, white pants with gold buttons connected with shiny gold chains running down the visible leg, and white jackets with the same gold buttons. A shiny black colonial coach trimmed in gold with four white horses also high-stepped and stopped behind the men on the black horses.

After the church bells clanged loudly three times, a handsome wedding couple came running down the cathedral steps, hand and hand. The bride and groom were laughing, each with brilliant white teeth and a copious amount of wind-blown black hair. The bride was dressed entirely in white and just before ascending into the coach, the bottom of her dress extending far out in all directions, the hoop seemingly lighted from within. A middle-aged man wearing black boots up to his knee, a crimson red topcoat with gold buttons and a black top hat, sat on a gold cushion holding the stirrups, stoic with eyes fixed front.

The entire affair was extraordinary. But with no phone to take a photo or video, and my wife preferring to watch than film with her phone—I think she was punishing me because of my grumpy behavior—I sank into deep melancholy, knowing I would never see such a spectacle again.

The following afternoon, sitting in a café at the western edge of the Jardin, we watched couples dance to live music from musicians standing in a white shell in the middle of the park. Though partially obstructed by leafy branches, we saw men of all generations dressed in cotton whites— even the sombreros were white—respectively asking women to dance. I saw no señorita or señora refuse; the partners methodically stepped around the band shell without expression. Our elderly waiter explained that the dancing occurs every Sunday since as far back as he could remember.

I gasped, "What a beautiful tradition."

My wife answered, "Yes. You can see customs like this all over Mexico. Too bad journalists never cover them; they only write about drugs, corruption, and violence."

I bellowed, "Indeed!"

I remembered my phone. I took it out of my waist belt, shook the phone violently several times, and quickly went through the dozens of possibilities again, thinking the shaking might do the trick. Thwarted at every turn, I sat and brooded, missing much of another cultural delight.

On the third night, as we walked down another cobblestone street lined with the usual ketch (e.g., handbags adorned with the ubiquitous face of Frida Kahlo), we passed restaurants with wonderful smells of moles and meats, and boutiques overflowing with bright colored rebozos, guayaberas, and hats of many colors and styles.

We reached a corner and debated about which restaurant to go back to when the faint sound of a brass band slowly grew louder. We turned to the vibrating foghorn sound of a tuba, the playful roller-coaster zip of a slide trombone and the recurrent boom of a drum only to see darkness, but seconds later, a couple emerged out of the night, looking somber. As I watched them move into the light, they were very short and had dark brown skin, and the woman wore a white wedding dress with many ruffles. The man was dressed in a rumpled black suit with a white shirt and thin black tie askew. They were followed by rows of men, women, and children of many shapes and dressed in different colors, coming out of the shadows, singing. A band of eight men and boys brought up the rear of the humble wedding party, holding brass-colored horns, a large drum, and a giant tuba that was bigger than the boy carrying it.

I mumbled, "What a shame. I could have taken a beautiful video. Maybe even made a documentary."

***

The following day, we were back on a bench facing the cathedral, listening to the sounds of church bells that inexplicably rang every 15 minutes. We watched two groups of 6 or so mariachis draped in white and gold with horns and guitars, strolling through the park, looking for someone who wanted to serenade a lover.

I was still tinkering with my phone.

Looking at the phone in my hands and losing patience, my wife called out to a young man walking by, "Joven!"

The young man stopped and turned. "Si señora."

"Would you mind looking at my husband's I-phone." As she explained my problem, I grew alarmed, thinking, here we go, this kid is going to take it apart, we'll sit here for an hour, and he'll have trouble putting the pieces back.

I stuck my stiff right arm toward the young man while glaring at my wife and loosened my grip on the phone.

The young man looked at both sides of the phone and, after turning the back of it toward me, he said in English, "You have a piece of gum covering the lens."

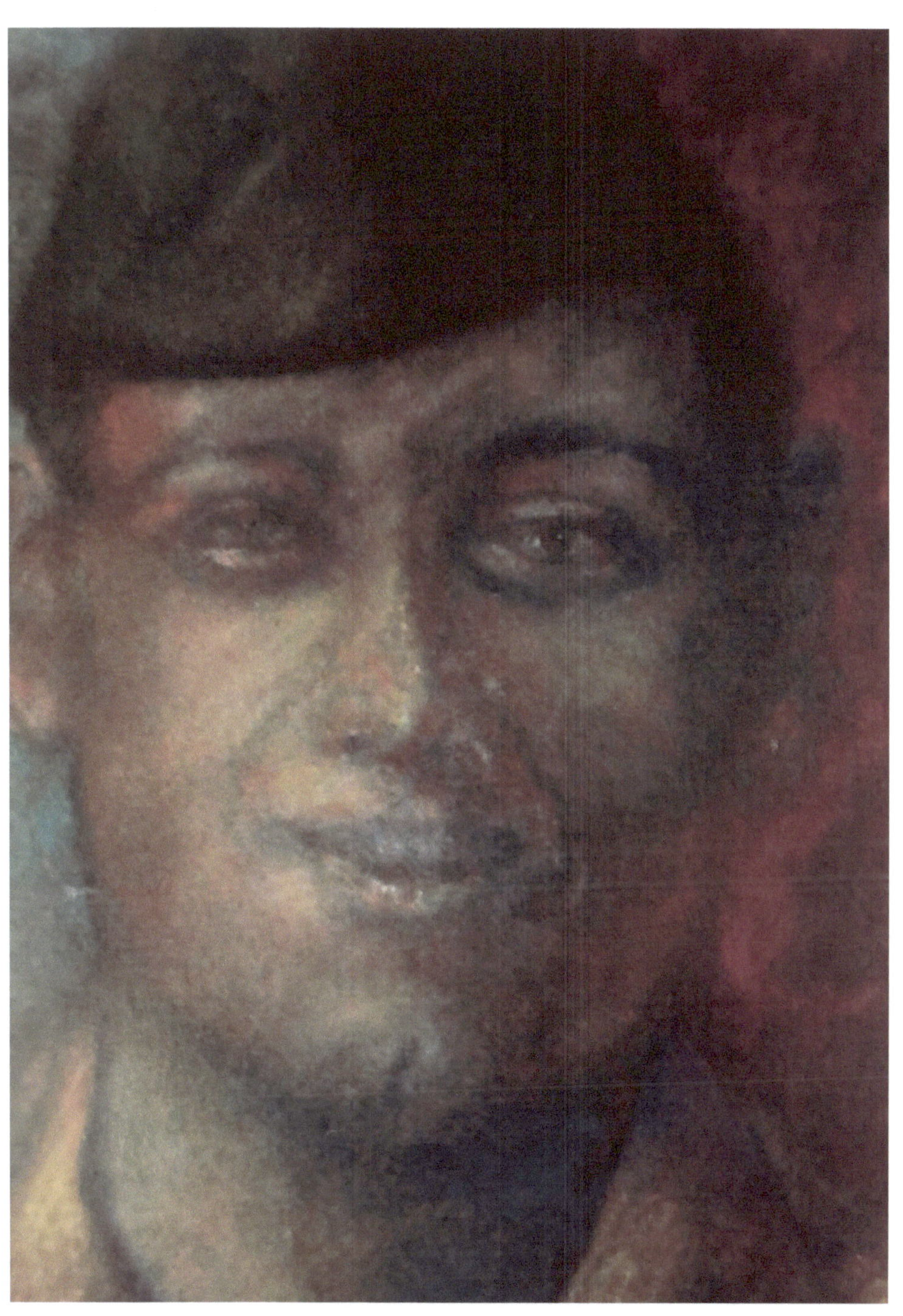

Rick Pringle
Vietnam
Private Collection

The Illegal Veteran

The six-truck convoy of supplies was slogging down Highway # 11, which stretched to the horizon, shimmering in the noonday heat. Two shirtless boys in dirty white shorts stopped kicking a soccer ball in the middle of swirling sand and yelled obscenities. At that precise moment, there was a deafening explosion. Harry Zapata's head and neck snapped backward.

After hearing the cries for a medic, Harry jumped out of the cab of the fourth truck and staggered forward with his M-16, trembling. A body was lying face first next to scattered debris, twisted steel with sharp edges, and a nauseating smell of oil mixed with burnt rubber. With his knees sinking into hot sand, Harry turned the soldier over, revealing a swollen red face with large blisters weeping clear fluid. The name Ford was sewn above a torn pocket. With his eyes quickly scanning the body, the medic saw sand-colored fatigues fused with black skin on the chest. The soldier was still except for wild darting eyes. Harry poured water from his canteen to cool down Frankie Ford's burns and injected morphine into an exposed upper arm. While applying a sterile Vaseline dressing on his friend's forehead, he heard yelling in Arabic and pings of bullets hitting metal. Harry pulled Ford's limp body under the nearest truck and, lying on his stomach, prayed the act of contrition.

The following day, Harry was evaluated for headaches in his base camp. A short, portly physician with a thick reddish-brown mustache matter-of-factly said, "Since you were three trucks removed from the explosion, you were merely stunned." The doctor handed Harry a plastic bottle of Tylenol.

After several days of worsening symptoms, including dizziness and relentless, pounding headaches, Harry got drunk. He stumbled out of the barracks, but after falling behind his drinking buddies on their way to midnight chow, he stopped in front of his company commander's headquarters. Swaying and squinting, Harry ripped off a poster of a smiling face atop dress greens encouraging soldiers to re-up, which was stapled in a kiosk. Screaming obscenities, he tore it into many pieces.

"Soldier!" Harry spun around and decked the intruder.

"Zapata, get up!" A helmeted MP marched Harry toward the scene of the crime. As he stood trembling in a cloud of smoke in front of a desk with a large ashtray full of cigarette butts, First Sergeant Moss looked up with his huge clean-shaven head, drooping jowls, and a bulbous red nose. Harry's eyes went back and forth from his boots to Moss's searing eyes.

Moss growled, "Do you know why you're here Zapata?"

With eyes downcast, Harry muttered, "I think I ripped up a poster out front First Sergeant."

"You think! And you slugged the chaplain! Do you remember that?"

Harry looked at Moss with widened eyes and pleaded, "No First Sergeant! I have no recollection of that!"

Moss rose with his palms on his desk, leaning forward, and shouted, "Well recollect this. The chaplain was trying to stop you. Less than a week! In 28 years, I've never seen someone fuck up so bad with such little time left. You're a descendant of Emiliano Zapata are ya? That ain't going to help you in the middle of Iraq son. You're screwed!"

Harry Zapata was dishonorably discharged for something he did not remember doing.

***

Harry dozed off into a dream. While mesmerized by a cactus with its arms lifted heavenward and illuminated by bright moonlight, he was pulled by his mother into the back of a long truck filled with the stench of unwashed men. Huddled men and boys were like shivering sardines; it was too dark to see their faces. Harry's tightly held on to his mother's hand. A loud blast threw him out of the truck. After looking up to a blistering, blurry sun with a throat full of burning sand, he tried to low crawl through mounds of foul-smelling yellow feces, gagging. Upon the sound of moaning, Harry looked to his left and saw slow moving streams of bloody flesh sloughing off of what used to be a face. The sewed in name above the shirt pocket was Zapata. The screaming woke Harry; he was soaking wet and violently shaking.

Harry took two gulps of vodka from a fifth sitting on his bedside table, curled up in a fetal position, and clutched a pillow. Within minutes, he glided into a relaxed state of mind and body. But with the blood alcohol level continuing to drop, the rock would soon roll back down the hill.

Harry lay alone on wet bed sheets smelling of urine, looking at the

ceiling. Sixteen years after returning from Iraq, he continued to suffer
from incapacitating headaches, dizziness, and hideous nightmares. Stoop
shouldered, he drifted from one menial job to the next. Alcohol helped
relieve these symptoms, but it became the source of other problems,
including broken relationships, long blackouts, and wicked withdrawal.

In agony from physical and mental torture in his head, Harry threw
his dishrag into soapy water, walked briskly out of the Tastee Diner
without saying a word to his boss, and took a cab to Parkland Hospital
in the Southwestern Medical District of Dallas. Following a thorough
history, neurological examination, and an MRI of the brain, a tall, thin,
brown-skinned physician with a white turban explained, "You sustained a
traumatic brain injury. The road side bomb rattled your brain, knocking it
against the walls of your skull."

Following further evaluation, Harry was given a prescription for
OxyContin, a psychiatric referral, and a follow-up neurology appointment.

After a morning opioid and vodka cocktail, Harry, smiling broadly,
went back to Parkland Hospital to keep his appointment with a
psychiatrist. Following a thorough evaluation, Dr. Pushkin— a middle-
aged woman with an oversized blonde wig, thick glasses, and a
Russian accent—said, "Your symptoms are due to post-traumatic stress
disorder, complicated by your traumatic brain injury." The psychiatrist
recommended, "A tranquilizer, don't drink, continue with individual
therapy with me, and PTSD group therapy." Harry got the sedative.

Standing in front of a bathroom mirror, Harry remembered when his
abundant black hair stuck up like a porcupine. With a bronze complexion,
thick lips, flat nose, and dark, intense eyes, one of his ex-girlfriends
thought he looked like Charles Bronson. But that was years ago. Not quite
40, he saw purplish sacks under each eye, and his hair was falling out. He
punched the mirror with his right fist, cracking it into many pieces, and
looked at bright red blood running off his knuckles.

However, shortly thereafter, Fortune finally intervened. Harry found
something safe that helped relieve his unrelenting headaches: marijuana.
And thinking about what the neurologist and psychiatrist said, at least
he knew what was wrong with him. He also believed that steady work
was possible as the sedative would resolve his anxiety, help with sleep,
and treat acute alcohol withdrawal—he only would only drink the nights
before a day off—thereby allowing him to return to work relatively stable.

For the first time in years, Harry was encouraged. With music blasting,
he drove to La Hacienda de Cortés, a fine dining restaurant in downtown
Dallas for a job interview. And while his resume was riddled with lies,
they were plausible. He nailed the interview with the Mexican owner

and was hired on the spot, which meant a lot more in tips than he was accustomed to in greasy spoons. Grinning at all the fine linen on the tables and the private party that awaited—a pint of cheap wine and potent weed—he was soon sitting in his beat-up, bright red Kia, slapping the steering wheel, and singing along with Aerosmith's, "Dream On."

Harry's alcohol and marijuana use was a balancing act that was working. Pain free, his take home pay for his first two weeks was more than he had ever made. Staying in a rooming house, after a month on the job, he began looking at newspaper ads for an apartment. He remembered being a straight A student in high school, before Iraq, and he thought about college to become a health care professional or journalist. And for the first time in his life, Harry entertained the possibility of quitting drinking and getting help to do so if necessary.

Ten minutes early and parked across from the large adobe-style restaurant that looked like the Alamo, with adequate, functional pain management, Harry was slapping his steering wheel to the beat of Queen's, "Another One Bites The Dust." But his optimism burst like a balloon; he turned his head left and saw a belly in a blue shirt. Without relevant legal or medical documentation in 2019, the joint Harry was smoking bought him a one-way ticket to Mexico.

***

Sitting on the deportation bus glancing out the window, seeing nothing but telephone poles wizzing by, Harry thought about finding some of his Emiliano Zapata relatives. He needed help, but with his great-great-grandfather having 19 children, there had to be scores if not hundreds of living descendants scattered about the tiny state of Morelos. Clinging to a frayed reed, he prayed that in finding family of the martyred hero— bonding with blood—he would find his true inner self buried among the wreckage of his past and perhaps a place where he belonged. He was seeking salvation.

A middle aged, obese man with the right part of his abdomen spilling into Harry's space was snoring. The man awoke, grunting his displeasure. After shifting his considerable posterior several times before settling in, he turned to look at Harry's profile, stuck his left hand under the stranger's chin, and said in Spanish, "My name is Fernando. Nice to meet you."

Harry clasped a massive, heavily calloused hand and responded, "Likewise. My name is Harry."

"I can tell by your accent you lived in Gringolandia most of your life."

Harry answered in torturous Spanish, "Yes. I came when I was a child.

And my relatives built roads and bridges in San Antonio; they went back and forth across the border without raising an eyebrow."

Fernando pulled out a sandwich that smelled of peanut butter from a brown paper bag, took a bite, and spouted, "Those days are long gone my friend." He asked while chewing, "Are you illegal?"

"Undocumented. The only thing I did was smoke a little weed. But my mother brought me here as a child. I'm a dreamer."

Fernando's head rolled back and he said through laughter, "Dream on my friend. Undocumented and smoking marijuna in Texas? You're on the one-way Trump express."

"Maybe. But on a more positive note, my great-grandfather was Emiliano Zapata. This deportation may be a blessing in disguise. I want to find my roots."

Fernando slumped in his chair and said, "Zapata you say? Sure. They will be calling you a Malinchista."

"What the hell is that?"

Fernando twisted his large upper torso so he could look Harry in the eyes. He explained, "Malinche learned Spanish and, acting as an intermediary between the Spanish Conquistadors and the Aztecs, helped Hernán Cortés."

"I know that. What does that have to do with me?"

"Malinche is the embodiment of betrayal. Malinchista is a word to describe a Mexican who promotes American culture over what is Mexican."

Fernando twisted his torso back around and resumed chomping on what was left of his sandwich. Harry looked at the side of Fernando's brown leathery face with white stubble.

Fernando, licking his fat fingers, said, "I wouldn't go around Zapata's old stomping grounds saying you are his descendent with that gringo accent of yours."

The bus arrived at an immigration facility in Laredo, Texas. Dozens—diverse in age, sex, and education, among other things—were herded into an overcrowded, hot room with bright light, where they sat on plastic white chairs for more than two hours. Dressed in blue jeans and a yellow polo shirt, Harry was drenched in sweat with the T-shirt stuck to his skin. An officer announced that two cardboard boxes on a table contained bottles of water and sandwiches. Harry grabbed one of each. He tore open opaque wax paper to find ham and yellow cheese stuck in-between two slices of stale white bread. He took one bite and threw it in the garbage.

***

The group was marched over the Juarez-Lincoln International Bridge to Nuevo Laredo, Tamaulipas. Heads hanging down with many in tears, they were met on the other side of the border by Mexican Immigration officials. One uniformed young man, with a black hair buzz cut and white framed glasses said, "Please sit and wait your turn."

A baby wailed in her mother's arms. The official shouted, "This is not our idea."

By the time Immigration let the caravan go, it was pitch black in Nuevo Laredo. Harry saw an ATM machine and while repeatedly looking behind him, withdrew 4,000 pesos from his savings account. Treading in darkness gingerly, he saw many men congregating on street corners and, surveying the landscape with an aching palpating throat, Harry watched moving silhouettes with glowing red dots floating before him.

Harry had nothing for his hammering headache. He went into a dimly lit cantina filled with loud ranchero music, walked straight to a bathroom stall, and put $3500 in pesos into his right sock. He walked out into a barroom filled with cigarette smoke and loud laughter and sat at the bar, next to a drunk with long black hair over his face, unsuccessfully trying to keep his head up.

After the third shot of tequila, Harry bought the drunk a drink, and he consumed two more shots mixed with beer in a thick glass mug. Looking straight ahead at a long line of booze bottles of many sizes and shapes, he became wistful, remembering standing at attention in basic training. Without a male mentor in his life, he craved and responded well to the military structure and esprit de corps. There was promise then. But after his brain repeatedly slammed against his skull and the betrayal by the only country he had known, there was only despair. Harry looked above the bottles and upon seeing his reflection, he finally liked what he saw: determined and fearless on his quest for the holy grail.

Walking out with a pint of Jack Daniels in his right hand, Harry ate three tacos carnitas on a paper plate from a street vendor, hailed a cab, and boarded a bus for Mexico City. He sat in the empty back seat, merely dozing as there were many people hauling large bags, getting on and off at numerous stops. After drinking a half of the pint of booze, he was able to sleep and transferred to an early morning bus to Cuernavaca.

Upon arrival, Harry bought three cheap white tee shirts, underwear, socks, three pints of Jack Daniels, and a white gym bag. He checked into a downtown hotel, sat up on a bed with the help of three pillows, laid off the booze, and watched a Mexican movie that he did not understand.

The following morning, sitting in an outdoor café with huevos rancheros and coffee spiked with Jack, Harry watched a short man with deep set eyes approach the table. Squinting, he thought the guide's cavernous lines running across his facial flesh made for an interesting face; its tread depth suggested wisdom born of suffering. It was 10 am sharp. Paco Reyes doffed his white straw hat, revealing short grey hair neatly combed to the right.

Wearing a thin, rumpled cotton white suit, business-like and polite in manner, Reyes sat down, sipped a black coffee, and agreed on a price for a full day tour, which included the towns where Emiliano Zapata was born, assassinated, and buried. Harry stressed the need to find some of his Zapata relatives. Reyes's only acknowledgment of that request was a slight nod of the head without making eye contact.

They walked through the large cement square under a canopy provided by large oak trees. In the middle of the square stood a two-times bigger than life-sized sculpture of Emiliano Zapata on a galloping horse. Atop sat a typical Mexican sombrero from the revolutionary period with its extra-wide brim and high-pointed crown. Zapata's iconic thick mustache curled down both sides of his lips. He was brandishing a machete in an out-stretched right hand. There was a quote on the base of the sculpture: "I'd rather die on my feet than live on my knees."

Harry followed his guide down a narrow cobblestone street to Reyes's car. The auto was an old, black Volkswagen Passat with several large dents, including on the passenger door. Harry took his pint of Jack from the gym bag that was strapped to his left shoulder, took a big slug, and got in.

Harry brought up being related to Zapata a second time, but Reyes kept his eyes on the road, identifying points of interest. The accent was one thing; Harry suspected Reyes also wondered about the relatively light complexion of his client. But he said nothing about his mother being raped by an Irish priest in a convent not far from where they were driving. While true, he had no desire to go there as his story already sounded a bit over the top.

Upon arriving in Cuautla, they exited the car and sat on a park bench in front of a 30-foot, copper-colored bronze statue of Zapata, wearing a long cloak to the tops of his boots, holding the barrel of a standing rifle on his right side. He was buried under the monument.

The guide concluded his lecture by declaring, "Emiliano Zapata and his men fought in support of the new revolutionary government, and he was promised that the land stolen from hundreds of farmers in Morelos would be returned. It was not. Zapata took up arms and held most of the state until he was set up, ambushed, and killed by Federales on April 10, 1919."

"100 years ago."

"Exactamente señor. 100 years ago."

Harry's headache returned with abandon, throbbing like a sledgehammer hitting his forehead. After seeing a pharmacy doctor and buying some OxyContin, he washed two pills down with what remained of his whiskey and returned to the bench. Sitting next to Reyes, Harry remembered standing at his mother's death bed in Army dress greens. He could see her facial bones pushing against her thin layer of wrinkled brown skin. Seeing her emaciated body with rapid and shallow respirations, he kissed his mother's cheek and whispered, "Don't leave me mamita linda. I have found a calling. I will make you proud."

Looking up at the stone face of his great-great-grandfather, soft glints of moonlight reflecting off the left side of his nose, mustache, and chin, Harry grimaced and growled, "How in the name of God did I end up like this?"

Still looking up with Reyes at his side, after the sedation swallowing up the headache, Harry declared, "Zapata's image is everywhere. A hundred years after his death, he remains a hero to the vast majority of Mexicans!"

Reyes snapped, "Si Señor!

Harry asked the guide to drive him to Anenecuilco, the town of Zapata's birth. Upon arriving, Reyes saw an old man sitting on a bench in front of a small grey stone house. He stopped the car and asked through the open window if there were any descendants of Zapata that lived in the town. Standing and pointing to an alley, the old man said, "Go to the last house. Ask for the lady."

After parking the car, Harry and his guide walked on a hard mud path, passing a dozen small stone houses painted lime green, cerulean blue, and white. There was a plowed field on the other side of the street, with a boy bent over dropping seeds from a burlap bag. They heard the sounds from a cow and chickens coming from behind the houses as they walked. A small black dog stood in their path unyielding, barking. The last house was a simple stone dwelling painted white and covered in twisting green vines. No one answered Reyes's knock on the door. They walked around the house to the back. Standing in the middle of a small, white wooden fenced-in yard was a huge Amate Amerillo tree, its thick Naples yellow trunk terminating in wooden roots above ground, twisting like snakes in all directions.

To the left of the tree stood a short, round woman, wearing a loose-fitting white cotton dress. She stopped hanging clothes and turned to look at the men. The woman had an oval dark brown face. In a soft voice without making eye contact, Reyes introduced Harry as the great-great-grandson of Emiliano Zapata.

With her chin elevated, the woman responded, "My name is Maria Luisa Zapata Luz. I am a great-granddaughter of Emiliano Zapata Salazar."

The woman shook hands with Harry vigorously but showed no emotion. Maria Luisa said she was too busy to talk, but since she had to go to Cuautla in the morning with her brother, they could meet in the park where Zapata was buried at 9 am. She added, "There are many of us" before turning around to resume her work. Harry looked at her grey hair pulled back into a long pigtail that fell to her waist and his throat ached. He walked out of the yard and down the mud path next to Reyes without saying a word; it was a purposeful walk as though he was marching.

They drove back to Cuautla in silence. Reyes parked his car on the edge of the square park. Harry walked toward the colossal Zapata—the epitome of order, honor, and moral clarity—stopped, and looked up at his forebearer with tears rolling down his cheeks

Harry pointed to a two-story building on another edge of the square, painted a dull yellow, peeling in many places revealing rust-colored stone. Cantina para los Valientes (Cantina for the Brave) was painted in red above the swinging brown doors. Harry looked at a cactus to the left of the doors with its arms raised. He yelled to Reyes sitting on a bench, "How about a drink my friend?"

They sat at a round dark wooden table with a bottle of Tequila and two shot glasses in the center. After downing a third shot—Reyes had waved off a second one—Harry said, "Zapata was a martyr."

The guide answered, "We believe so. Absolutamente!"

Hoisting another shot above his head, Harry thunderously proclaimed, "Paco, thanks to you, I am finally home. After downing that fourth shot, Harry shouted in muddled Spanish, "Maria Luisa Zapata is my blood. Emiliano Zapata is my blood!"

And for the first time, Reyes acknowledged Harry's noble lineage. "I am happy to be of service Señor Zapata."

Harry closed his eyes. He remembered some of the brutal ordeal crossing the border to the land of milk and honey; the fear of being caught, the punishing dessert, stuffed in a truck filled with the stench of scared men, followed by an image of his mother, squeezing his tiny hand while standing in front of a small white bungalow in East Los Angeles, proclaiming, "Son, no more fear. No more running. This is our home."

Harry ordered a large plate of a variety of tacos—chicken, steak, and pork—on corn tortillas garnished with onion and cilantro. Reyes ate two tacos, whereas Harry had 4 of the remaining 8. With red and light green salsa all over his white tee-shirt, he continued to talk of his good fortune—

finding family—throughout the meal.

As Harry turned to summon the waiter for the check, Reyes heard two men talking at a nearby table. One of them growled, "Que blasfemia! Puta Gringo! Malinchista!"

Reyes knew that the men heard every word of Harry's Spanish with an unmistakable American accent. Turning slightly to his left but keeping his eyes downcast, he only saw a pair of red cowboy boots with pointed toes curled up under a table.

Reyes heard the same voice from behind as he and his client walked out of the cantina. He walked briskly. Harry exclaimed from behind, "What's the rush Paco?" Reyes did not turn around or respond until they reached the central part of the square, amongst a throng of people. He informed his client about what had happened. Harry rubbed his chin while examining the faces in the crowd.

Reyes walked Harry across the square. They passed the Zapata statue with moonlight reflecting off the cone of the sombrero atop the massive bronze man cloaked in darkness, to the Hotel Morelos. He shook Harry's hand and said, "Good Luck my friend. Stay with people and you will be O.K." The guide turned and walked away, but he suddenly stopped at the sight of two men masked by the shadows of the night. Reyes's eyes moved down the silhouettes to cowboy boots with pointed toes curled up.

The guide turned around and walked into the hotel. He stood in the lobby and looked at the back of Harry standing in front of a hotel clerk. He hollered, "Señor Zapata, I will see you at 8:45 am, and be there with you to meet your relatives."

Harry turned around and answered, "Thank you Paco. I really appreciate that. I'll be in the lobby."

After cancelling an early morning appointment and staying the night with a nephew, Reyes went to the Hotel Morelos the following morning. The hotel clerk, with an ashen face and quaking voice said, "Señor Zapata left the hotel last night. He said he was having a very bad headache. I watched him walk across the square and go into the cantina. About an hour later, I heard shouting and saw two men dragging the gentleman into the alley."

Reyes took a deep breath, shuddered, and asked, "Where is he?"

The clerk answered, "He's in Cuautla Hospital. I walked across the square and looked into the alley next to the cantina. I watched the gentleman being savagely beaten with fists and boots, particularly about the head. I heard a man screaming; '¡Malinchista! ¡Hijo de la chingada!' Someone called for an ambulance. No one called the police."

***

Dr. Miguel Navarro, a neurosurgeon, dressed in light green surgical scrubs and cap, walked into the hospital morgue, a large white room with bright light. Harry Zapata lay on a silver gurney, under a white sheet in the middle of the room. Dr. Navarro pulled the sheet up and then down, revealing multiple black and purple contusions on a bloated face. The eyes were swollen shut.

Standing stoically on the other side of the gurney was the old woman that Harry met the previous day, wearing the same baggy white cotton dress. An old man with a long, sad face and thick grey hair parted in the middle, dressed in white cotton shirt and pants, stood next to the woman, head bowed. He stepped forward, lifted his head and said, "This man is a Zapata. We will see that he is properly buried in a cemetery with our people."

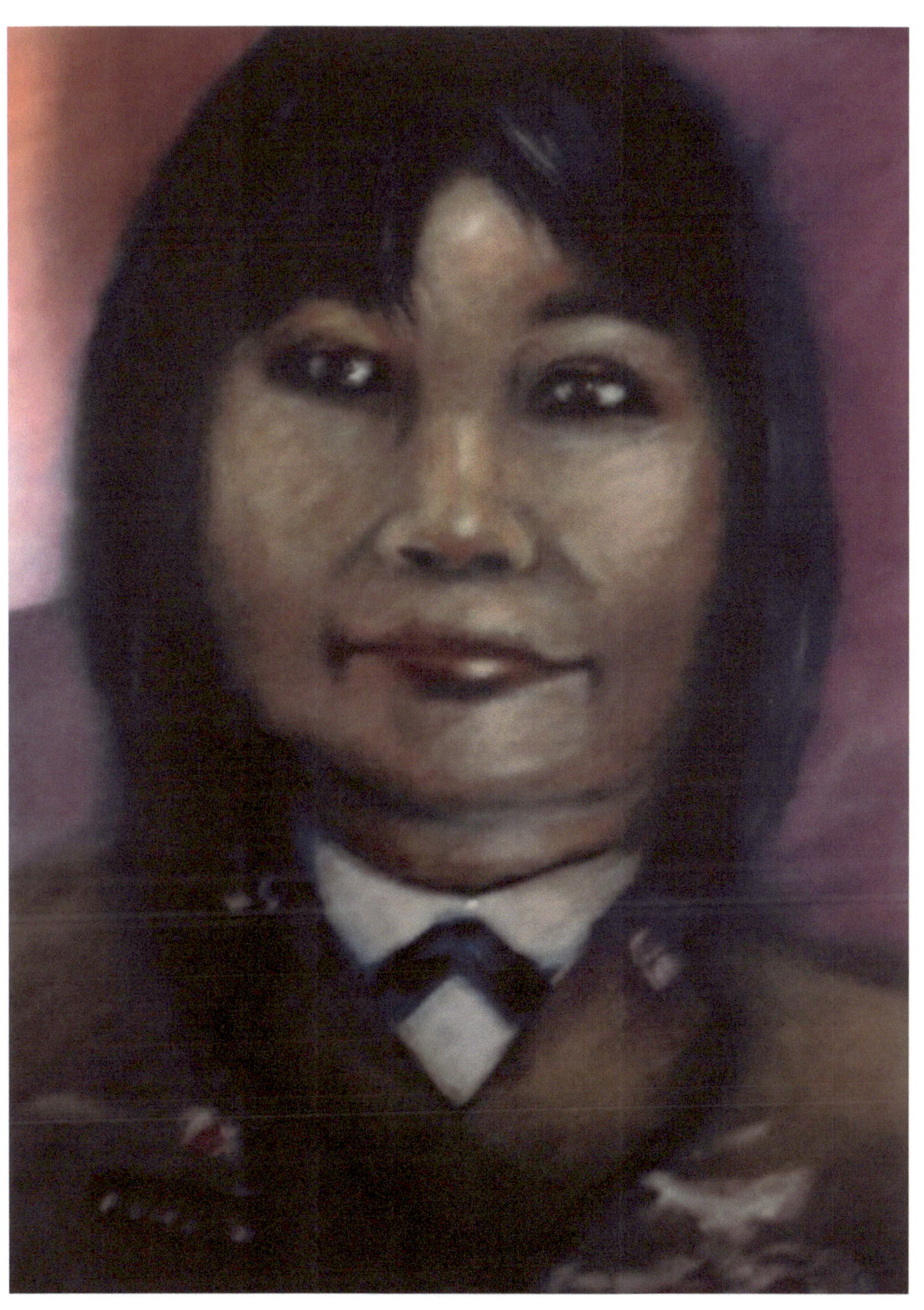

Tammy
Iraq
NYC VA Regional Office Museum

Dreams Shattered

"... if dreams die
Life is a broken-winged bird
That cannot fly."
-Langston Hughes

Peggy Stark, a bespectacled short, chubby, and annoyingly cheerful nurse brought the new medic into the Emergency Room (ER). She announced, "Tom, Sonny, this is Terrance Wallace."

Wallace was dressed in crisp olive-green fatigues and cap, fresh from Supply. He was a tall, skinny teenager with bulging hazel eyes and a long neck with a huge Adam's apple. Fidgety, Wallace could not maintain eye contact. After a handshake with Tom Mulligan, he grumbled, "I don't know how I ended up here. I volunteered to kill gooks."

Sonny Larson lowered his large head on a thick neck and mumbled, "What an asshole."

Wallace made a left face and snarled, "You're the asshole fat fuck. Whose side are you on?"

"Larson responded, "All victims of this senseless battle."

"Nose-to-nose, like a manager arguing with an umpire, Wallace shouted, "Senseless? That's exactly why we are losing this war."

The nurse deftly slid in-between the combatants while pleading, "Now boys, let's not get off on the wrong foot."

After Wallace stomped out of the ER, Mulligan said to Larson, "Holy shit! You can tell in a few seconds there's something wrong with that guy."

"You're right. I've got to play it cool. I'm going home in two weeks."

***

The petite Vietnamese girl sat in a white plastic chair for the last of her 3-hour sessions, motionless as Sonny Larson molded the heavy Indian red clay. Leaning against a tall locker, Tom Mulligan marveled at how such massive hands had the dexterity to reproduce the fine features of the girls' face with pouting lips. Bent over between two bunks with the clay head on a flat table, studying his muse, Sonny captured the sweetness and vulnerability of the petite 16-year-old Tam.

Sonny Larson was 6 foot 2 and weighed over 250 pounds. He always looked like he had just dragged himself out of bed in his faded, baggy yellowish-green fatigues. His dirty blonde hair was never combed, sticking out every which way, and he usually had light brown stubble on his fat face with large, sagging jowls. Brown-reddish smears of clay were all over his hands, face, and Army green tee shirt.

Mulligan watched Sonny apply the last thin layers of wet clay to complete Tam's diminutive nose and high cheekbones.

They heard distracting thumps getting louder. Private Terrance Wallace, marching through the middle of the barracks in his spit-shined black jungle boots, came to a halt. He turned to his right and spat, "So you're a faggot too fat boy?"

Larson never took his eyes off his model.

***

The 3rd Mobile Army Surgical Hospital (MASH) was in the middle of the Mekong Delta. While the withdrawal of the U.S. 9th Infantry Division was underway, the choppers kept bringing the wounded, including young American and Vietnamese soldiers, Brown Water Naval personnel, occasional Viet Cong, and Vietnamese civilians of all ages. Army personnel stationed at the 3rd Surg included scores of medics at any given time; they were among those that had guard duty on a rotating basis.

Sonny Larson kneeled in the guard tower before the pitch-black night, hearing the distant sound of whirling blades of cobras and buzzing mosquitos in his face. With the aid of a night lens on his M-16, he was riveted by streaks of white light emanating from the gunships. He remembered running with his younger brother waving sparklers with glee in the darkness of his back yard in his early teens on the 4th of July.

Larson glanced at his watch, stood up, and turned to look over the compound of eight long rectangular, rain-streaked, brownish grey wooden barracks, four on each side of a wide sidewalk with rectangular patches of green in-between, lit up by spotlights. In the distance lay the hospital made of corrugated steel of a silver hue, with its rows of wards jutting out on each side of a long corridor. It looked like an airplane with multiple wings ready for takeoff. To the left of the hospital, a chopper hovered over a landing pad with a big red cross. There were dark figures with two stretchers moving toward the chopper. Larson thought how everything looked so neat and orderly from above, in sharp contrast to the blood-splattered walls within the ER.

Larson spotted his relief, Tom Mulligan, moping toward the guard tower. Mulligan was medium in height and wiry with neatly trimmed black hair and mustache. Strapped with his M-16, he carefully climbed up the ladder, pausing on each rung. Looking up at the opening of a huge basket, he said to Larson's eyes peering down, "This reminds me of climbing up to my boyhood tree house. But this ain't no game."

From Mobile, Alabama, Larson greeted Mulligan's ashen face with a bass-baritone southern drawl. "It ain't nothin. Just don't shoot any good guys or fall asleep."

Mulligan responded, "I've been up here already. I'm fine as long as I don't look down."

Larson laughed while looking down at the ground and teased, "At least you can pick off the enemy if they overrun the place, coming up the ladder. Keep shootin, one VC at a time."

Mulligan quickly walked around the basket while looking out and excitingly said, "They'd probably throw a grenade up here."

"Throw it back."

Mulligan took his M-16 off his shoulder while exclaiming, "What the hell are medics doing up here anyway?"

***

Terrance Wallace sat alone at one of a score of long tables in the Mess Hall, as far from everyone as he could get. Mulligan and Larson were eating breakfast four tables over from the newbie. A hard rain was pelting the metal roof. Mulligan whispered, "Did you hear Wallace is a security guard?"

Larson answered loudly, "Yeah. He's a clumsy, shitty medic, so he got the boot."

Mulligan answered, "That's a good thing."

Larson shot back, "Yeah, but that weird fuck having a weapon all the time? That's a bad thing. My last guard duty's tomorrow and I have to relieve that punk."

Wallace slammed his tray on the table, the noise reverberating through the Mess Hall. He stood up and walked across the room. Standing behind Larson and glaring down at the top of his head, he growled, "You got Vega's shift, so you relieve me in the morning fat boy." He turned and slowly walked out.

Mulligan shrieked, "You're gonna let that go?"

Larson calmly drawled, "He's fixin for a fight. I can wipe the floor with that obnoxious jackass. But I ain't gonna rock the boat. A final guard duty and I'm short 12 days and a wake-up baby!"

"Yeah. Stay away from that nut case. He told Vega his dream is making a difference in the war. The fucking guy just got here. I also heard that his father's a lieutenant general."

Larson got up from the table and said, "Oh yeah? Maybe that's why he's so fucked up."

***

In one of the 8 two-story wooden barracks, Mulligan's bunk was next to Larson's. Their two bunks were walled off by tall lockers. There was an aisle running through the middle of the barracks, separating another cubical with two bunks. Mulligan, having just come off a grueling shift in the ER, lay in his bunk, staring at the ceiling, trying to forget putting a burnt Vietnamese boy in a body bag.

Sonny Larson lumbered through the middle of the barracks; he had a wide gait that yielded to no one. With his considerable posterior sinking into his bunk, he looked at the supine Mulligan.

Larson lit a joint with a match and took two hits before stretching his right arm toward Mulligan, saying from the back of his throat through sucked in and held smoke, "This is good shit man."

Mulligan sat up and took two hits.

Larson said, "Hey man, dig my art portfolio." He opened a large, thick book of photos of sculptures he had made. The photos were in plastic sleeves, two to a page. As Larson gently turned each page, he said most were done in clay and then cooked to make them bronze.

Mulligan cooed, "Yeah man. The people and animals look real. Like that running white horse. Beautiful."

Larson leaned forward and proclaimed, "Now dig my abstract work!"

Mulligan blurted out, "What the fuck is that?"

Larson rolled his eyes with a big smile. "I'm prouder of them because they come from my head. Not just looking at something and making what I see. You can take a photo if that's all you want to do. Some of them are made with found objects. They are put together using all kinds of materials."

After looking at the abstract art, Mulligan said, "I like the ones of people and animals a lot better. You can see you're really good. I don't know what the fuck I'm looking at with this other shit."

They both burst out laughing.

***

The following day, Mulligan and Larson finished their 12-hour shifts in the ER after putting a 21-year-old American soldier in a body bag. Lawrence Johnson, a gunner in a cobra, had sustained gunshot wounds to his right shoulder, abdomen, and left thigh. He died of a blood clot that went to his brain. While holding the upper half of the bagged body, Larson cried out to no one in particular, "What did this kid die for?"

Tom Mulligan, a 19-year-old son of fervent Catholics, came from Meadville, a small city in Northwestern Pennsylvania. The Mulligan family had a long history of fighting for their country, including Tom's uncle James, who was killed in action on the island of Bougainville in the South Pacific during WW II. He was 26 years old. Tom believed the Vietnam war was about stemming the flow of communism and keeping the South Vietnamese free. But Larson's rants against the war seemed to make sense. Mulligan was confused and conflicted. There were many like that. Mulligan laid on his bunk and stared at a stationary lizard on the ceiling, its throat seemingly pulsating in perfect time to the rising crescendo of "White Rabbit" by Jefferson Airplane, drifting in from a few cubicles away.

Directly across from Mulligan, looking down while lacing his boots, Larson announced to all within earshot, "Eleven days and a wake-up!"

With eyes closed, Mulligan's brain began to slow down and he drifted to a Meadville golf course, barefoot with pants rolled up, picking up balls from the bottom of a creek, but within seconds, he was jolted awake by a girl's terrified, high-pitched screams.

Wallace was standing in the cubical across the aisle, framed by the rows of tall footlockers, towering over the tiny, terrified Tam, with the barrel of his M-16 a few inches from her head. Then he crouched down and put the barrel under her chin. In a deep voice, Wallace growled, "Hey Baby San. I'm going to blow your head off for doing a shitty job on my boots. You charge too much money for number 10 job."

With tears streaming down her face, Tam's response was a fearful, unintelligible babble.

Mulligan sat up and said to Wallace, "Hey man, put the weapon down." As the girl fell to the floor, Wallace turned and pointed his M-16 at Mulligan's head, with the barrel less than a foot from his left temple. Wallace shouted, "Mind your own business. I'll blow your fucking head off." Tom froze. No one moved.

The barrel began to move again, pausing to center on Sonny Larson. Still sitting on the edge of his bunk and lacing his jungle boots, Larson lifted his head and said, "Quit fucking around Wallace. You're not supposed to leave the guard tower."

Wallace shouted, "You're late Larson! Get your fat ass in gear!" Two popping sounds immediately followed, before the weapon hit the wooden floor with a thud.

A silver wristwatch flew off Larson's wrist and suspended in mid-air before smashing on the floor. There was a thumping sound of Wallace's boots hitting the floor as he ran out of the barracks.

Larson's screams of pain and fear were only interrupted by gasps for air. Within seconds, the cubicle was a bloody mess.

Mulligan rushed over to a geyser of bright red blood from what looked like Larson's head. He was still sitting on the edge of his bunk, and his arms were bent at the elbows, one on each side of his head, rocking back and forth, screaming. Mulligan gently pulled Larson's arms away from his head and saw a gaping right forearm wound with gobs of thick, bloody flesh and a shooting stream of bright red blood. There were many pieces of bone fragments amongst the ripped muscle and tissue. Below the wound, a piece of bone stuck out of Larson's skin like the tip of a tusk.

Mulligan ripped off his Army green tee shirt and applied pressure on the wound; the moving crimson soaked up the green. Calmly, with his left arm, he stretched and pulled a thin white towel from the base of the bed and used it to tie a tourniquet above the wound. Larson had lost an awful lot of blood, but the pressure bandage on the forearm helped stem the flow and the tourniquet stopped it cold.

Cookie Rosario, practically a midget with an overgrown Fu Manchu moustache and mop of black curly hair, suddenly appeared in the cubical shouting, "Did he get hit somewhere else? Look at the pieces of his watch on the floor."

Mulligan responded, "Yeah. Look. He got nicked on the right wrist."

Felix Fontaine arrived with a silver gurney. Mulligan, Cookie, and Felix struggled but finally got the heavy, howling Larson on the wheeled stretcher. Mulligan picked up the broken watch and put it on the gurney beside Sonny. It was in three pieces.

Cookie, one of numerous cooks at the 3rd Surg., gently placed his hand on Larson's left shoulder and said, "You're going to be O.K. Sonny. We stopped the bleeding in time."

Mulligan added, "They'll patch it up and you're going home a little early Sonny."

Larson finally stopped screaming, probably from sheer exhaustion, but the blood had drained out of his face. With his head turned to the right, Sonny's eyes were fixed on the three pieces of his silver wristwatch; the round face of the watch was still ticking.

***

A few days after the shooting, Mulligan was sitting at a table in the EM club with a can of cheap beer, when Rosario walked in. Cookie picked up a wooden chair, turned it around, straddled it with his chin resting on the back of it, and solemnly said, "They had to amputate Sonny's right arm in Japan."

Mulligan responded, "I'm not surprised. The two bones in his forearm were shattered. Jesus. Short 11 days."

"That ain't all I heard. The CO said Wallace hung himself at Long Binh Jail."

Mulligan drank the last gulp of beer. Crushing the empty can with his right hand, he bellowed, "He was just a scared kid. And there was something mentally wrong with him. Somebody should've caught that."

Cookie, looking at the crushed beer can on the table observed, "And his old man being a general didn't help any."

After lighting a cigarette, Mulligan blew a few smoke rings and while watching them dissipate, softly said, "And a couple of dreams shattered."

Cookie asked, "What dreams?"

"The kid wanted to make a difference, whatever that meant. He probably wanted to impress his father, the general."

Cookie lifted his chin from the back of the chair and asked, "And Sonny's dream?"

"He wanted nothing more than to make sculptures."

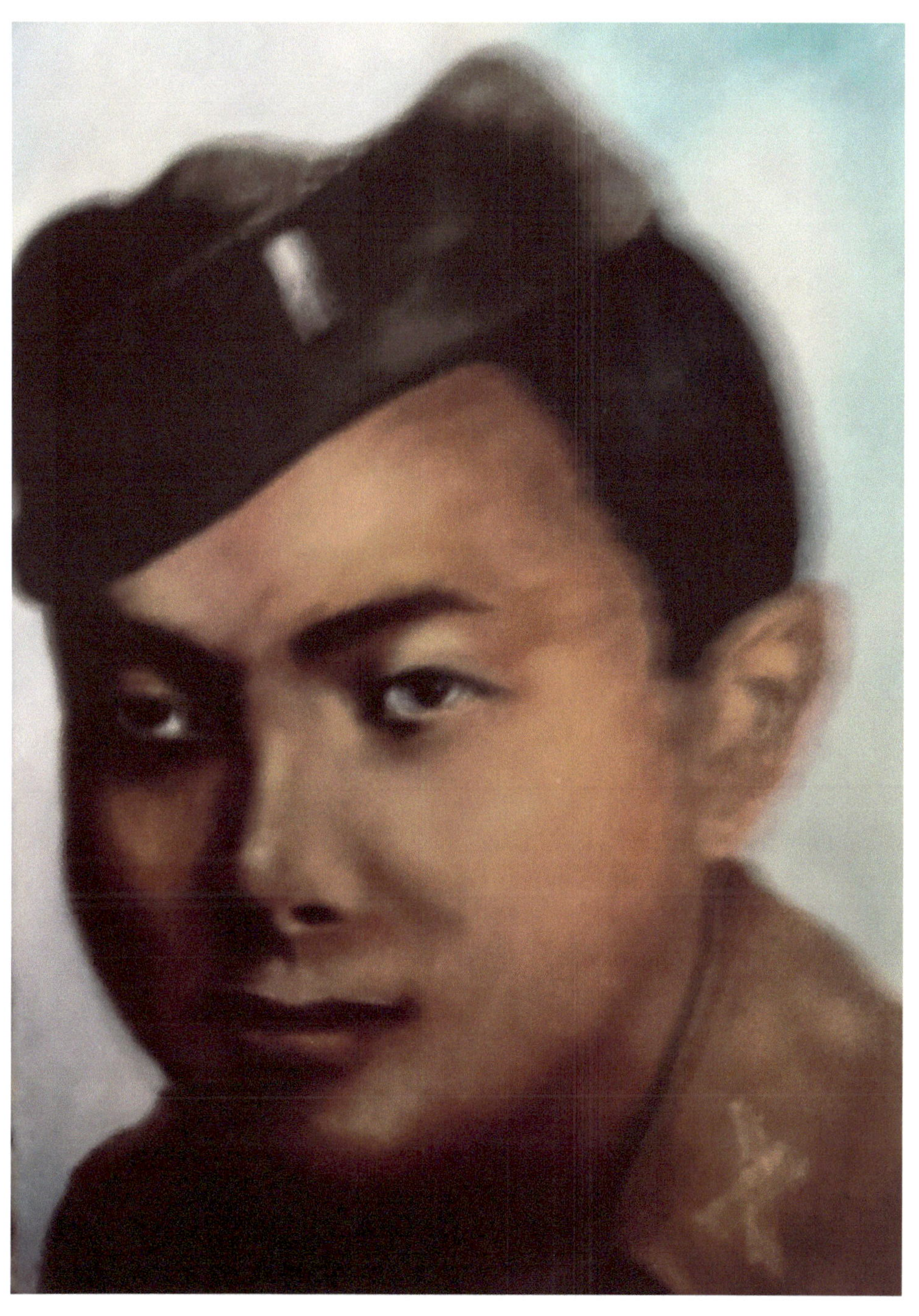

Lee
WWII
Buffalo VA Regional Office

Careless Disregard For Those
Who Shall Have Borne the Battle

Frank Russo cursed at his tall, thin image in the mirror as the third attempt to knot his tie failed. Tremulous, he looked at his wife Lois with a pleading expression. Standing in front of the same large rectangular mirror in their hotel room applying red lipstick, she smiled and said, "Let me do it; you're shaking like a leaf."

After Lois reached up and tied a perfect knot in her husband's brown tie, she picked up her lipstick and resumed applying it to her lips. Still standing beside his petite wife, Frank said to her mirrored image, "I'm a nervous wreck. I'll be glad when this is over and we're back home. This is costing us a fortune and it's a big waste a time."

Lois frowned at the listlessness of her grey hair as she slid her lips across each other and dabbed a Kleenex on her lower lip to remove some excess red while mumbling, "Why do you say that?"

Bent slightly forward due to disc disease in his lower spine, Frank walked a few steps and sat on the edge of the end of the bed, still looking at his wife's mirror image as she lightly applied powder to her checks and snub nose from a compact and answered, "Because Gallagher pretty much said so. Something about the numbers not adding up to a 10 percent rating. Jesus Christ. I'm nearly deaf!"

Lois turned and looked down at her sitting husband wearing a pout. She bent over and kissed a small round bald spot on the back of his otherwise healthy head of grey hair, sat next to him on the bed, slipped her right arm under his left arm, and rested her head on his shoulder while saying, "But you came here to make a point, didn't you? About the injustice of how the VA doesn't compensate the hearing loss of combat veterans?"

Frank answered through clenched teeth, "You're damn right I did. I'm not holding anything back either!"

Lois stood up and picked up her black purse with a long horseshoe strap, the color complementing her black sweater, bright yellow pleated skirt, and low black heels. She turned as Frank slowly rose and, still looking in the mirror, pulled the ends of his suitcoat on both sides down and straightened his tie by making the knot tighter.

"Leave the tie alone Frank. You look fine. We better get going. It's a ten-minute walk to the VA and it's already twenty to 11."

Frank turned and faced his wife. "Yeah. And I'll bet it's hotter than hell already in this swamp of a city. Let's go and get it over with."

Frank Russo combed his silver-grey hair back and parted it in the middle of his head. In addition to his bent over frame, he walked with a pronounced limp on the right due to severe arthritis of the right hip. Dressed in a light brown cotton suit, white shirt, and dark brown tie that was slightly askew from his nervously pulling on it, he held out his tremulous right hand for his wife of 37 years; she took two quick short steps while extending her left hand and jointly, they followed the veteran's Disabled American Veterans representative into the hearing room. Lois pulled the chair out for her husband and sat next to him on his left side, the representative sitting to the veteran's right; all sat in front of a long rectangular table of dark brown wood. They were waiting for judge who would conduct the hearing and decide the veteran's appeal.

Frank's service representative was 63 years old, a World War II veteran with over 25 years-experience representing veterans. Leo Gallagher was a large man in height and girth with a thick Boston accent. He had a large head with thinning white hair and a deep booming voice that filled the room. After they met him in his office the day before the hearing, Frank said to his wife, "Gallagher's voice will rattle the rafters." There was an instant bond because the representative had also been in combat in the European theatre, and he exuded confidence. Lois Maloney Russo did not like his gruff manner initially, but by the end of the hour-long session in Gallagher's office, she appreciated his humor, particularly after he talked about his penchant for brooding with a dancing gleam in his right eye and quoted the poet Yates on being Irish.

While Leo Gallagher was hunched over reviewing his notes, Frank and Lois Russo looked around the large room. Behind an elevated 10-foot-wide table with a thin silver microphone in the middle, hung photographs of Harry Walters, the Director of the Veterans Administration; and Ronald Reagan, president of the United States; there was part of an unfolded American flag in the background of each photo. A large drooping American flag stood in the corner, left of the podium. There were four soft dark brown leather chairs where the veteran, Lois, and Gallagher were seated. A glass pitcher filled with water and 4 clear tall glasses sat on a silver tray in the middle of a long rectangular dark wood table.

While his wife was inspecting her husband's hair and suit, Frank continued to look around the room. There were four tall, narrow windows on his right; he watched young men and women in business suits filing up and down "I" Street, many carrying briefcases. The windows were shut tight but that did not prevent the frequent muffled sounds of car horns seeping into the room. On the wall to the veteran's left hung patriotic framed prints, to include George Washington heroically standing in profile in a small boat with his men crossing the Delaware; and an iconic photograph of Abraham Lincoln with his beard and mussed hair; the quote underneath the latter photograph read, "To Care For Him Who Shall Have Borne The Battle, And For His Widow, And His Orphan."

While it was already 92 degrees at 11 am on this August Monday morning in Washington, D.C., the hearing room at the Board of Veterans Appeals was comfortable with central air, but Frank Russo was sweating. He could feel the wetness under his arms and using a handkerchief, he repeatedly wiped rolling beads of perspiration off of his forehead.

Lois turned and placing the palms of her hands on her husband's cheeks, gently turned his head to face her and with her fingers extended from her right hand, combed her husband's abundant silver-grey hair off his forehead toward the back of his head. Frank whispered, "I wish I could calm down. I only got 2 hours of sleep last night."

Lois, kissing her husband lightly on his forehead, responded, "It's O.K. honey. You'll be fine."

Lois folded her hands on the table in front of her and looked around the room, pausing at the photographic portrait of Reagan. She thought it was remarkable that her husband and the president still had such abundant hair. A fly landed on the edge of one of the water glasses. Lois shooed it away.

At exactly 9 am, Judge Harold Slocum entered the room carrying the veteran's thin light brown cardboard claims file. Dressed in a blue pinstriped suit, white shirt and blue and red striped tie, the judge, short and stout in stature with a thick white mustache and wearing horn-rimmed glasses, stepped onto the elevated podium, and sat in a large black chair behind a long rectangular table. After a rattling cough and clearing his throat, he tapped the long, thin silver microphone in front of him with an extended right index finger, which triggered a loud, high-pitched piercing noise that shot through Frank Russo like an electric current.

"Good morning Mr. Russo. My name is Harold Slocum. I will be conducting this hearing. Before I swear you in, I need to go over some preliminary matters with your representative. Mr. Gallagher, the only issue before the Board of Veterans Appeals is entitlement to an increased rating for bilateral hearing loss, currently rated zero percent. Is that correct?"

"That is correct Judge Slocum."

"Will there be any testimony besides the veteran?"

"Yes sir. The veteran's wife will be presenting testimony."

The Judge responded, "All right. Mr. and Mrs. Russo, please stand and raise your right hands. Do you swear to tell the truth, the whole truth, and nothing but the truth, so help you God?"

Frank and Lois answered in unison, "I do."

"Please be seated. Mr. Gallagher, do you have an opening statement?"

"Yes sir. The veteran served honorably in the United States Army and was assigned to the 37th Tank Battalion of the American 4th Armored Division during World War II, which was the spearhead of General George Patton's Third Army. It was during that time that he was exposed to acoustic trauma as the result of his manning heavy artillery in a Sherman tank. The veteran was exposed to heavy weaponry fire on a nearly daily basis for two months. His hearing loss has worsened over the years. He retired early from his job as a truck driver, in part, because of his service-connected hearing loss and tinnitus."

Frank and Lois were distracted by the buzzing of a fly that landed on the edge of the glass again.

Mr. Gallagher continued, "The hearing deficit and constant ringing in the ears caused significant job impairment. If I may Judge Slocum, I would like to ask the veteran a few questions."

"Please proceed."

"Frank, tell me your duties while with General Patton's Third Army; specifically, your duties while inside one of the Sherman tanks in the 37th Tank Battalion."

"Well Mr. Gallagher, my hearing loss and ringing in the ears began after I was exposed to all the noise from high-velocity 76 mm M1 guns inside a Cobra King tank. It was constant explosive noise hours at a time, sometimes on a daily basis over a two-month period. I joined the Army and volunteered for combat duty I was only 18 years—"

The judge interjected, "Excuse me Mr. Gallagher. The veteran's acoustic trauma during service is not at issue here. In other words, the VA has already established that the veteran's hearing loss was caused by noise exposure during service. The question before the Board on appeal is—"

The veteran interrupted, "Noise exposure? The noise was deafening, constant." Frank balled up a fist and hit the table with it while saying, "bam, bam, bam, bam—on and on—lasting many hours at a time over a period of many weeks. It blew my ear drums out."

The judge responded, "Yes sir. That is not in dispute. The point I'm making is that the issue before the Board is the current status of your hearing loss. That is, the proper rating based upon the current severity of your hearing impairment."

Frank became visibly tremulous—you could hear the tremor in his voice—and he was sitting on the edge of his seat with both of his palms and forearms pressed against the table, ready to rise. "I can't understand how it was rated zero percent in the first place."

The Judge glanced at his notes in his hands, shuffled some papers, cleared his throat and stated, "The VA rates hearing loss on the basis of applying the results of your audiological examination to the rating criteria; medical facts; specifically audiological test results applied to the law. It's pretty straight forward. It simply comes down to the numbers we have. And the range we look at is the normal conversational range. Compensable ratings are warranted based up certain levels of hearing loss in the normal conversational range."

Frank Russo's face felt burning hot and his heart was beating fast; he could hear and feel it beating in his ears. Lois looked at her husband and extended her right hand and placed it on his left forearm and squeezed it.

Frank became limp as he turned his face to his left to acknowledge his wife's concern, but he stiffened as he turned back facing the judge and declared in a loud voice, "I don't mean to be disrespectful sir, but I got two problems with what you just said. First of all, the test is like I'm in a sound proof booth. There is no background noise. That's not reality. You don't go through life in a sound proof booth."

Frank turned to his right and looked at Leo Gallagher. His representative sat back in his chair and with a nod of his head and a flick of his right wrist, encouraged the veteran to continue with his testimony. Gallagher thought Frank was making an important point better that he could.

"The second thing is I got high frequency hearing loss. As I understand it, the kind of noise exposure I'm talking about—very loud noise from large weapons—causes high frequency hearing loss. There are millions of combat veterans walking around with this kind of hearing loss. And when you say normal conversational range, that leaves out a lot of people. My wife has a high-pitched voice. I can't hear her half the time. I can't hear my grandkids. That's my normal world!"

"I understand sir."

"Do you? I also have ringing in my ears. Day and night for 40 years and that started during combat. And they give me 10 percent for that. It seems to me that—"

Judge Slocum interjected, "I do not have that issue before me Mr. Russo. I'm looking at your file. I see that service connection is in effect for tinnitus. I can refer the matter back to the regional office. That is, I can raise the issue of entitlement to a rating in excess of 10 percent for tinnitus and send it back to the San Francisco Regional Office for adjudication. But I—"

"How do you rate that? Is there a way I can get more than 10 percent for that? It's constant in both ears."

"I do not have that issue before me Mr. Russo. You have not filed a claim. However, I can refer it back to the regional office in San Francisco and they will adjudicate the claim. But your current rating of 10 percent is the maximum evaluation for tinnitus."

"Why am I not getting it for each ear? The constant ringing is in both of my ears."

"Ears cannot be rated separately for tinnitus. That is, the maximum rating allowed for tinnitus—by law—is 10 percent. But as I said, I cannot make a determination on that question because the issue is not on appeal. It is not before me. But I will refer it back."

"What's the point? You just said I can't get more than 10 percent."

Lois placed her right hand on her husband's left forearm again and squeezed it hard.

Frank pulled his arm away from his wife's hand, rose to his feet, steadied himself with his right hand on the table and said in a quivering voice, "So I'm going through life not being able to hear my wife or my grandchildren and a lot of other things, and I've got this noise in my ears—in my head—that tortures me constantly, and I'm rated 10 percent for all of that?"

The judge snapped a stern look to the veteran's representative and said, "Mr. Gallagher, I have six hearings scheduled today, so I'm going to ask you to address the matter at hand: entitlement to a compensable rating for the veteran's hearing loss."

Gallagher sat up straight and answered, "Yes Judge Slocum. Please sit-down Frank."

Frank did what he was told. He felt the perspiration popping up on his forehead and streams of sweat rolling down his back. Lois poured a glass of water for her husband. His throat was dry and he looked at the half glass of water, but like someone with Parkinson's disease, he feared he could not hold the glass without spilling the water.

Following a series of questions from Gallagher and answers from the veteran about how hearing loss adversely affected the latter's employment as a truck driver, including retiring early because of his hearing loss and tinnitus, Lois Russo offered confirming testimony.

After whispering her intention into her husband's left ear, the veteran's wife rose and meekly inquired in a high-pitched voice, "Judge, my husband has a lot of trouble sleeping. He has nightmares and some are about the war. It has gotten a lot worse since he retired last year. Is there something that can be done about this?"

Judge Slocum responded, "You are raising an issue of entitlement to service connection for post-traumatic stress disorder or PTSD. I don't have that issue before me either. I cannot address issues that have not been adjudicated by regional office. However, I will refer the matter back to the San Francisco VA Regional Office for adjudication."

Lois asked, "But how long is that going to take? It took three years to get this point where we are sitting now."

The Judge bowed his head, pretending to look at the claims file, raised his head and said, "I don't know how long it will take ma'am. I have no control over timeliness at the regional office. It depends on the backlog of cases in San Francisco."

***

Leo Gallagher summarized his argument, to the extent one could be made under existing law. Frank and Lois each thanked him for his effort while shaking hands. They turned and walked out of the hearing room, down a long hallway and onto the street. They crossed "H" Street and walked into Lafyette Park in silence. There were many office workers in shirtsleeves sitting on park benches eating their lunch out of brown paper bags or white Styrofoam boxes with white plastic knives and spoons. Frank and Lois stopped to look at a statue of Andrew Jackson on a rearing horse atop a massive stone pedestal in the middle of the park. The sun was bright and hot in the noon-day, cloudless blue sky. Lois pulled a pair of sunglasses from her purse and put them on. She looked through the park to the front of the White House, partially obstructed by the leafy branches of trees, and remembered standing on Pennsylvania Ave. facing the White House with her parents when she was a little girl.

With her head tilted slightly right toward Frank, looking wistful, Lois said, "When I was 12, my parents brought me the this very spot. It was spring and it was cool. We walked past the east wing of the White House all around to the back. There was a softball game on the Ellipse. We took a tour to all the monuments."

Frank looked around the park at the young people sitting on the benches—they all looked very young—and turned to his wife and said, "No one is talking to anyone else. I don't know how they can sit out here in this heat."

After walking to the front of the park, which bordered Pennsylvania

Avenue, with their backs to the front of the White House, they stood on the south edge of the park reading a six by six-foot cardboard sign with "Stop the Bomb" handwritten with a black magic marker on the upper half of the sign and two large photographs on the bottom half. A middled-aged woman of no more than 5 feet tall stood next to the sign wearing a threadbare navy-blue pea coat and a red scarf over a bee-hive hairdo despite the oppressive heat and humidity. She answered yes to Frank's question of whether she was the author of the anti-war statement. The woman launched into a diatribe about the atomic bombings in Hiroshima and Nagasaki, pointing to two large pictures near the bottom of her sign that showed Japanese bodies scattered on the ground that appeared burnt and dead. Some looked like children.

Frank and Lois walked east on Pennsylvania Avenue toward 15th Street, noticing a very high steel fence painted black that extended around the front lawn of the White House with the bars on top terminating with sharp gold points. Frank observed, "There are cameras and security all over the place but some nut always tries to go over it every year or two."

Lois stopped walking, turned around, took off her sunglasses, and looked back at the White House shimmering in the heat. After gazing at the park across the street they had just left, she said in a voice tinged with melancholy, "Remember when we brought the kids here? Kennedy was president."

Frank grunted his concurrence, looked back toward at the woman with the large sign in the park, and said, "He was assassinated a few months after that."

They passed the U.S. Treasury building; a massive structure of stone painted white with many monolithic columns and pilasters and a sculpture of the first Secretary of the Treasury, Albert Gallatin standing in colonial dress on a pedestal in front of what Frank thought looked like a Greek temple. They made a right turn on 15th Street and walked toward their hotel but decided to stop on the way at the Old Ebbitt Grill, a Washington institution that was a block from the Hotel Washington.

A waiter brought Frank and Lois to a table near one of the four bars in the huge restaurant. Frank asked for a table away from the noise and they were brought to a booth. He looked at his wife and then up to the waiter and said, "This placed is mobbed."

The waiter was tall and thin with spikes of dirty blonde hair, held in place by gel and pale blue eyes. While handing menus to the couple, he said through a laugh, "We are always busy but believe it or not, a few hours from now, between the dinner and happy hour crowds, there will be twice as many people. Can I start you folks off with a drink?"

"Frank looked at the waiter's black bow tie and said, "A bottle of Budweiser.""

Lois answered, "Just water please."

Frank followed up with, "I think we know what we want. I'll have a cheeseburger with fries."

Lois, glancing at the menu, looked up at the waiter and responded, "I'll have the same. Medium rare. But no fries. Can I have the house salad instead?"

"Certainly ma'am."

After obtaining additional information on the order, the tall smiling waiter withdrew. Frank looked at his wife sitting directly across the table. "He looked like a teenager."

Lois answered, "They all look like teenagers."

Thinking about the woman with the sign in Lafyette Park, Frank softly said, "After surviving the Battle of the Bulge, they were going to send me to Okinawa in August 1945 to fight the Japs. I would have been a dead man 40 years ago if it wasn't for Truman dropping those bombs. They say we would have lost at least 100,000 men invading Japan. The Japs would have fought to the last woman and child."

Lois nodded her head in agreement as the waiter set their drinks before them.

Frank poured his beer in a tilted tall beer glass and took a sip. "I thought about my father today during the hearing. Don't ask me why. He was a fisherman on the east side of the bay. He knew Joe DiMaggio's father. They were both fishermen from Sicily. His son became my hero growing up. He was the best ballplayer I ever saw."

After taking a sip of water, Lois said, "I remember him. He was such a good-looking man. Didn't he marry Marilyn Monroe?"

Frank ignored his wife's question and responded, "He enlisted but never left the country. He played baseball with troops here at home to build morale, I guess. I enlisted and volunteered to fight. I saw men die all around me. One was decapitated in front of my eyes. I've had nightmare and ringing in my ears ever since. It ain't right. Something ain't right."

"No. No, it's not right honey. But I was proud of you today. You stood up and—"

"What? I can't hear a word you're saying Lois."

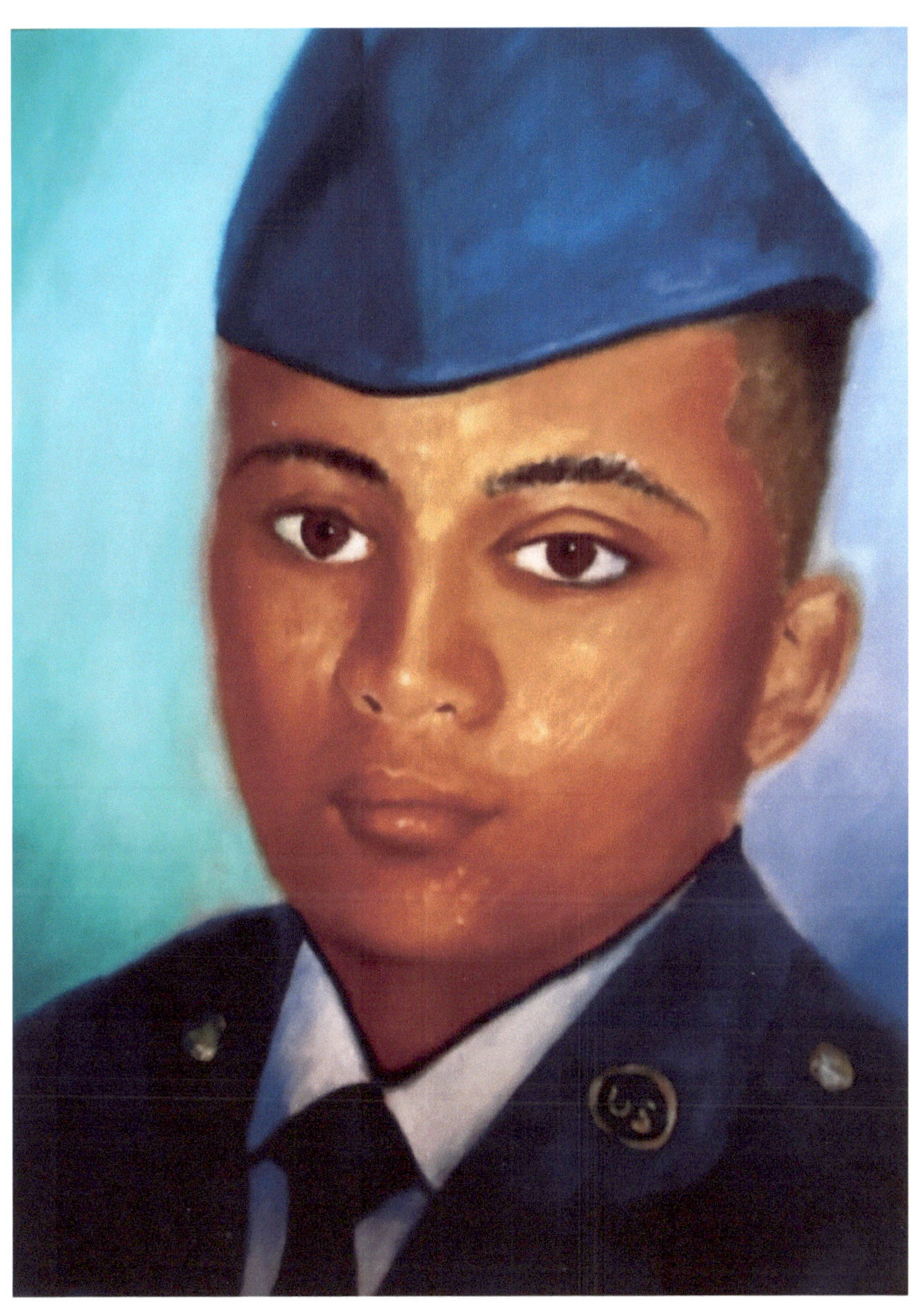

Wilfredo, Age 21
Iraq, KIA,
Buffalo VA Regional Office

The Necessity of Hitting Bottom

After calling 911 for an ambulance to my home more than 20 miles away, it was a maddening ride out of downtown D.C., racing up Connecticut Avenue, weaving in and out of traffic. I was overcome by a second wave of panic at the thought I might get pulled over, and flying down Old Georgetown Road to Suburban Hospital, where my son lay with what I feared was a life-threatening head injury. Sitting in my office moments earlier, the call I received from his teenage friend Howard was jarring enough—"Eddie fell and hit his head on the cement patio"—but following my gasping, "Put Edward on the phone," my son's incoherent, sluggish ramble sent me into a tailspin. Stunned, I knew that lethargy and mental confusion following a head injury were bad signs. I feared the worst possible scenario: brain swelling, coma, death.

Sweating profusely in balmy weather with my white shirt sticking to my back, I parked erratically and illegally in an employee parking lot and ran into the emergency room (ER). A nurse unsuccessfully tried to calm me down and ushered me into the waiting room. While gently placing her right hand on my left shoulder and leading me toward a chair, she said, "The doctor will talk to you shortly."

I was too jittery to sit; rather, I paced back and forth in the waiting room without making eye contact with the several people sitting in chairs for what seemed like hours until a young physician, evidently forewarned by the charge nurse that I had repeatedly pestered her for information, walked into the waiting room. Dr. Monaco, short with a black handlebar mustache that hung over his upper lip, dressed In light green scrubs including a soft cap over a mop of curly black hair, extended his right hand and after shaking my right hand while introducing himself, said, "You can relax Mr. McColl. Your son's head injury was minor but we had to pump his stomach. He was grossly intoxicated."

"Drunk?"

"That's right. You can go in to see him now. He's still a bit groggy, but he's responsive."

With mouth agape, I was relieved but nevertheless astonished. Acute alcohol poisoning—falling down drunk—had not occurred to me. My son was 15 years old.

I stood at my son's bedside; Eddie was lying on an ER gurney with the guardrails up, in-between walls of dull green-colored curtains pulled forward from the wall to ensure privacy. While holding on tightly to a corner of a white sheet pulled up over his face covering everything except part of the right side of his head, including his rapidly blinking eye, he acknowledged me with a muffled, "Hey Dad," but his eye jerked left and locked on the ceiling fan above him. After I began speaking, he twisted his body toward the wall away from me, burying his face in a pillow.

"How are you feeling Eddie?"

His response was a smothered, "Awful. Embarrassed. Sick to my stomach."

"Let me see your face."

Eddie rolled over, turned his head toward me, and slowly pulled the sheet off his face with his right hand. There was a two-inch laceration on the left side of his forehead that was sutured, a circular area of dark blue-purple with a yellowish border the size of a silver dollar surrounding the suture site, and what looked like a smear of black paint between his left eye and eyebrow. His pale blue eyes were wet and bloodshot.

"Well Eddie, it doesn't look too bad. But what the hell happened? Where did you get the alcohol?"

With downcast eyes, Eddie answered in a barely audible voice, "Howard's brother gave us a bottle of vodka."

"Why did you drink so much of it?"

"It was stupid. I don't know what I was thinking. Sorry Dad."

"I'll be having a talk with Howard's parents. What's more important is that you learn from this. The doctor said you could have died from acute alcohol poisoning. In other words, you came close to overdosing. And you know our family history of alcoholism. Almost everyone on my side. It killed your uncle Sean at age 31. And I gotta tell you; normal drinkers don't end up in ERs getting their stomach pumped."

Looking into his vacuous eyes, it was evident that my counsel went in one ear and out the other.

***

That was the first of many episodes of alcohol intoxication that I know of. (With the most predominant symptoms of alcoholism being denial, rationalization, and minimalization, alcoholics are unreliable historians. That's a nice way of saying notorious liars.) Drugs would eventually enter the mix and a parade of lawyers, judges, and probation officers would follow, surrounded by frequent parent-teacher conferences and occasional parent-principal meetings. I used what leverage I had; Edward completed alcohol and drug treatment programs of increasing intensity or confinement: out-patient, in-patient, and a half way house. It was a rocky road indeed and shortly after his 19th birthday and washing out of his first semester of college—he didn't show up—and after forging a check for $500—we have the same name—I gave him an Army enlistment or out-the-door ultimatum. He chose the former.

Eddie drifted from friend to friend over the next several weeks, wearing out his welcome and eventually running out of friends. After he called and asked to meet, I sat across from my son at a local McDonald's. Sitting in a corner booth with a Baltimore Orioles baseball cap pulled down over his eyes and holding on to a twisted "handle" of a large dark green trash bag filled with his clothes, he tearfully begged me to let him come home. It was heartbreaking as the tears rolling down his cheeks were real, but I knew this was a critical juncture in his life and with our relationship, and I had to summon the strength to resist caving as I had thrown up my hands and surrendered numerous times during a variety of crises. While wavering, a friend's question and observation proved helpful: "When you rescue your son, are you doing it for him or you? When you do that, you are preventing him from hitting his bottom and without that bottom, he'll never ask for help."

Edward enlisted in the Army shortly thereafter and the 3-year stint did him well, all things considered. Given his lifestyle, perhaps it saved his life. And knowing he was not roaming the streets with his crew or in a car driven by someone impaired by drugs or alcohol—far less likely anyway—I could sleep.

***

I was a single parent throughout my son's teenage years. Most often it looked and felt like we were roommates rather than father and son. Edward on his cell phone passing me in the hall; me looking at his back as he sat lotus-style on the carpet playing Nintendo or watching Bevis and Butthead on TV. Meals on the fly. While I tried (and not hard enough in retrospect), dinners at the table with conversation became increasingly rare beyond the mid-teens"

Teenagers can be persistent and exhausting; I remember having an image of tag team wrestlers but unfortunately for us, there was no one else to enter the ring. I was able to hang tough facing an onslaught of emotional pleading on the question of an automobile. I don't think my son would have survived like two of his friends had not—he was that kind of drinker—so I'll give myself a much-needed pat on the back for that.

We did watch an occasional movie together during Edward's teen years, although it dwindled down to a precious few a year as he went from animated Disney flicks to action films with numerous explosions and bodies flying all over the screen. Once, after returning from blockbuster with three movies in hand, he asked, "More boring black and white movies Dad with only talking?"

(I hark back to my early and mid-teens, my family of 7 gathered in the living room, prone on the carpet with my face propped up with elbows and chin in the palms of my hands, watching a Sunday night line-up of Bishop Sheen, Liberace, and Ed Sullivan. There's something to be said for such routine—predictability, stability—although being force fed the good Bishop after he swooped into the room with his cape like Loretta Young, terrorizing us with his list of mortal sins drawn on a blackboard that meant eternal damnation—a list that included eating meat on Friday—was a bit over the top.)

There was baseball; I was Edward's coach for 4 years of Little League, which guaranteed being together in my car to and from practices and games, and a common interest—a bond of baseball—evolved as it did with my father. I tend to minimize such healthy interactions because it felt like they were swallowed up by the unpleasant and occasionally alarming manifestations of my son's drinking and drugging escapades.

When I was a teenager, my parents were old and tired and there were too many of us so the odds were good that any misbehavior would slip through the cracks of their rather lame defense. You think about such things when you end up on the other side of this scourge. I only had one child and was more astute about drug and alcohol abuse culture and the warning signs of dependence than the average parent. As a consequence, a continuous cat and mouse routine emerged with me trying to stay one step ahead, ready to pounce on or intervene or block an impending disaster. But you can't foresee everything like sneaking out of the house in the middle of the night through a bedroom window, with the door-bell jolting me out of a sound sleep, finding a cop at the door with my 16-year-old son and his friend sheepishly limp with their heads hanging after they were pulled over in my car during a joy ride. Thereafter, I slept on the couch with my keys and wallet under my pillow on weekends. But it was whack-a-mole time as there was always something that I couldn't have possibly anticipated rear its ugly head.

Sometimes I wondered whether my son wanted to get caught. I found a bong behind the couch made with a plastic coke-a-cola liter bottle with a white tube coming out of the side fused with a flame. Or the sophisticated smoking pipe from Morocco that was almost in plain view in his closet. The latter warrants some explanation.

I went with a group of people on a tour to France, Spain and Morocco for 3 weeks and brought my 16-year-old son with me. We were on our own in the Medina of Marrakesh, with a guide I initially did not want but could not shake; I write initially because the medina was an incredible maze to a degree that I might still be in there but for the pestering guide. After pausing to browse in one of hundreds of tents with exotic wares laid out on fine fabrics of many colors, my son picked up a bronze piece not much bigger than my fist that looked at first like a lantern, the kind you would rub for a Genie. But it looked suspicious. I smelled an opening and sure enough: Hashish! I said to my son, "No way Eddie; I know what this thing is used for and I think you do too. He persisted but finally relented to my unequivocal push-back.

Lying on our hotel beds that evening, I told him the story of "Midnight Express" where an American traveling in Morocco (it was Turkey), got caught with a joint (I didn't remember how much he had)—and was thrown in jail for many years. (I didn't remember how many, but I suspected no more than 2 years.) I concluded by warning, "You could end up in a horrible prison getting beat up and raped after being caught at the airport with the burnt grounds of marijuana or hash in this thing, which is what I just smelled now!"

I felt assured that my dramatic lecture made the right impression on my son.

A few months later, following the discovery of another bong in our living room (under the couch), I inspected the entirety of my son's room. After rummaging through a pile of clothes on the floor of his closet, I found the bronze lantern. He went to considerable trouble to go back through the maze to buy it and smuggle it out; my dire warning hadn't fazed him. Holding the lamp in my right hand, I was struck still. I stared at it and smelled the opening. I shuddered.

***

Standing at our long rectangular living room window with the back of my left hand's fingers moving the curtain to the left, peering out into the black night, my attention heightened every time a silhouette emerged under a street light or was fleetingly illuminated by a passing automobile headlight. Teenagers all seemed to dress the same back then: baggy pants falling off their bottoms, ball caps pulled down over the eyes, doing the gangsta walk. "Is that Eddie? No. I think that's him. No."

A white van pulled into the plaza parking lot across the street from our home; it looked like my son's friend Mike's van. It parked and I watched and waited. No movement. I suspected they were smoking dope. I quickly dressed, jumped in my car, drove into the parking lot and circled the van. Finding tinted windows increased my suspicion. I wondered if there was drug dealing inside. I thought I could make out my son by the shape of a head and shoulders but while circling and squinting, I slammed into a tall lamp pole with the light up high and at the end of a silver arm that curved down. I jumped out and surveyed the damage while exchanging quick glances at the van. An old man with a full fuzzy white beard emerged from the van. He cried out, "Are you O.K.? Do you need any help?

I yelled back, "I'm fine. Thank-you. Just some minor damage here."

The white beard hollered, "You seemed to be quite interested in my van."

After mumbling a few obscenities, I shouted, "I thought I recognized my friend's van. Sorry about that."

"No problem. Be careful."

After raising my right arm with an open hand acknowledging the old geezer's concern, mortified, I quickly jumped in my car and drove the short distance to my driveway, sat, and hyperventilated. Then this sudden realization—some call it a moment of clarity—came into focus: I can't stop trying to rescue my son regardless of its futility without help. Regarding Eddie's bottom, I don't know what it will take or when it will happen if at all. But the good news is I know I've hit mine.

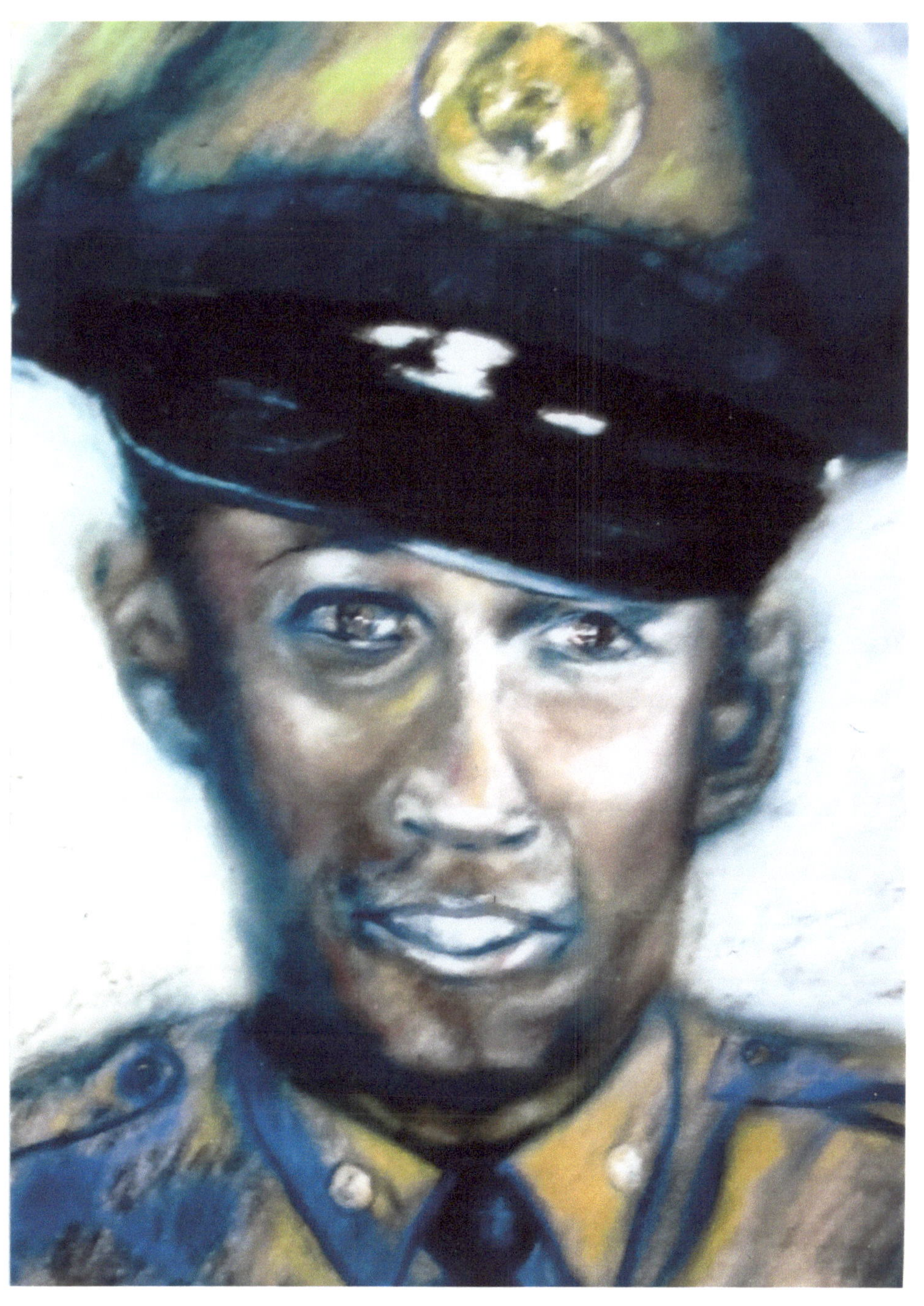

Vernon Williams
NYC VA Regional Office Museum

The Drunken Suit and the Bag Lady

It was late November 2002, and cold—that dark grey cold that descends upon the concrete city, accompanied by an icy, piercing wind, with swirling dead leaves in its wake. I watched expressionless mannequins in black suits and ties with briefcases on conveyer belts every morning. I was one of them. Bluster and rage galore raise the temperature, but it is inside the stone and marble. People rarely speak to one another outside the walls.

I was assigned to an anti-terrorism unit at the Department of Justice and was under the wing of one of the lawyers that wrote policy memoranda addressing the question of whether certain interrogation techniques were torture. After reading a memo on interrogating suspected terrorists, I was confused. I walked into my boss's office, keeping a respectful distance from his desk. Jacob Miller was 6 foot, 6 inches tall and weighed over 300 pounds. He stood up and waddled to the middle of the room. With glasses atop thinning silver-grey hair, he leaned into me and barked, "There is no ambiguity Rogers. No technique is torture if the detainee is not going to die."

I looked up and meekly asked, "You mean unless the suspect thinks he's going to die?"

Mr. Miller leaned further with my back was against the wall—think LBJ—and said, "No Rogers. Not just thinking he's going to die. We are only over the line if the terrorist is going to die."

Miller, gutturally laughing with ripples of fat rolling through his large abdomen covered by a thin white shirt ready to bust its buttons, added, "Between you and me Rogers, let's call it the breath on the mirror test."

In Miller's defense, this was only 14 months after 9/11, and we thought we were going to get hit again. Still, I was uncomfortable with the logic, especially as I had graduated from law school less than a year earlier and believed in constitutional niceties like the 4th amendment.

✳✳✳

I stopped in my favorite downtown bar for happy hour, a few blocks from work. The Fox and Hounds British Café was quite lively after 5 pm on a Friday with scores of dull suits and pantsuits. I was wearing my new charcoal grey suit with a dark blue, pinstriped shirt; solid powder blue tie; an expensive black wool top coat; and a fedora of the same color. The excitement of the nature of my work and being on Pennsylvania Ave., Ave., between the Capitol and the White House had waned considerably, replaced by a nascent philosophical conflict. Happy hour was an oasis where booze and laughter washed away such concerns. I often found interesting people to talk to (albeit not so fascinating the following morning when I threw their business cards into the trash).

The Fox was elegant, especially the long L-shaped bar with a shiny black Formica top and a huge mirror that ran the length of the bar. I could hear the tinkling of piano keys and singing from the larger room full of tables, but most of the revelers were at the bar, three-deep. Four young bartenders in red vests and bowties did their best to satisfy the Fox's thirsty customers. There must have been a thousand booze bottles. The blue lighting was dim, which I found alluring. Tasty tidbits, like spring rolls and small, triangular pieces of pizza were always part of the happy hour fare, laid out in orderly rows on a table adjacent to the bar.

Arriving at 4:30, I was able to get a stool at the small part of the L, thereby ensuring that I could see almost everyone in the room. I liked listening to the slow crescendo of chatter, reaching its pinnacle by 7 pm. I spotted an attractive bobbing blonde head in the crowd. Being well lubricated but not yet wobbly, I made my move, drink in hand. I had a nice jag going, but I inexplicably passed on the appetizers, so the booze rushed through the stomach lining into the bloodstream and flooded my brain, thus overwhelming my memory sensors. I have no idea if I talked to the blonde or anyone else.

The next thing I clearly remember is standing on the corner of K and 14th streets, a few blocks from the Fox, after 2 am, emerging from a 6-hour blackout, without my topcoat and hat. My car was in a closed parking garage—that turned out to be a blessing—and my keys were in my coat, but there was no money in my wallet or pockets. I knew I hit several bars after the Fox, but I only remembered scattered moments like flickering flashbacks of cloudy faces.

I didn't know where my coat was. I had no way to get home and did not have a credit card for a hotel. (With a night of serious drinking on the horizon, I always left my credit cards in my room out of fear that I might buy the bar a drink or get mugged.)

As I stood with my hands in my pockets shivering and moaning, an old woman pushing a shopping cart filled with clothes paused in front of me. Her name was Helga. She was probably about 65 years old. She wore a red scarf and two thick coats; the outer one was orange plaid. I still remember some of her face; she had very deep set, small dark eyes; a snub nose; a prominent chin; grey bangs on her forehead; and pale white skin with red patches and flaky scales. Helga had many thin wrinkles radiating out from her eyes and mouth. She squinted as she talked. Her voice was very high and squeaky.

As I approached, I said, "Good evening Ma'am. It's such a cold night. I'm new in town."

Without turning her head, Helga squeaked, "Mind your own fucking business."

"Sorry. I was just trying to be polite. I lost my car keys and money. I'm freezing to death. I have never been so cold."

She turned her head toward me, softened a tad, and whispered, "Are you a drunk? Only drunks are out at this time of night."

"No. I'm not a drunk. I mean I had a few drinks, but I'm a lawyer with the Department of Justice."

The woman abruptly turned to her right and began pushing her shopping cart west on K Street. She had a pronounced limp on the right. I caught up with her and said, "I didn't mean to startle you Miss. I'm not an agent. I don't investigate anyone."

Helga stopped walking, but she kept her hands on her cart. She did not look at me. I said to her profile, "I only write memos on how to investigate terrorists."

With arms stiffened, she pushed her cart faster; I had to run to catch up to her.

"Look. I'm just a low level, boring lawyer who is looking for a place to sleep. I have no coat or money. I think I was robbed."

"You think?"

"I was robbed."

"Is that how you got all that blood on the side of your face? You have blood in your ear."

"Blood?"

I carefully palpated the side of my face and saw no blood on my fingertips. I thought the lady was seeing things. But touching the top edge of my left ear revealed tenderness and bright red blood on the tip of my forefinger and my ear canal was filled with crusty crimson blood. There was a laceration on top of my ear; I had a blurry image of getting hit with the back of a hand from a guy in a ski mask, but this was the least of my concerns. I would soon have acute alcohol withdrawal symptoms and the temperature was below freezing; either calamity was potentially lethal. I needed booze to stem the tide of shaking to pieces in mind and body, and I considered asking the lady for a coat from her cart.

I pleaded, "Is there a homeless shelter? There must be a shelter for people such as you."

Helga got as close to me as she could, her face screwed up with rage. She slowly pronounced each word, striking the air in front of my nose with her index finger for emphasis, "What do you mean by people such as me? You're just another striped suit with a superior attitude."

"Look Miss, I meant no disrespect. I would ask the president of the United States the same question if he pulled up in his motorcade. I don't want to die out here in the street. I'll never survive this cold."

The lady's facial muscles relaxed and in a lower voice she answered, "There's a shelter. But I wouldn't go there. You wouldn't catch me dead in there. They rob people. They will take that suit of yours right off your back. That pretty blue shirt and tie too. I have a warm place to stay a few blocks from here. There's enough room. Follow me."

As I walked behind Helga hunched over while pushing her cart, I thought she must be an eccentric rich person. How else could she live within walking distance of the White House? I had read about such things. I knew that real estate in the D.C. area in the direction she was going was very expensive, especially after she made a left on 18th Street and then a right on Pennsylvania Ave. I watched her dark silhouette hunched over, pushing her cart toward million-dollar townhouses in Georgetown. Exhaling, I felt a sense of relief, albeit it was tempered by the oncoming onslaught of withdrawal.

I vaguely recall Helga stopping on a corner of Pennsylvania Avenue, somewhere in the 20s. She pulled out a pint of Kessler's whiskey—-cheap rot gut—and I took a couple of sips. Perhaps they were gulps, which would explain getting hit in the gut with a heavy purse. Helga must have become incensed at the two big gulps as she swung her bag that weighed a ton. I'll bet she had a few pints of booze in that purse; it knocked the wind out of me. Bent over, covering my head like a boxer and gasping for air, I pleaded for her to stop.

Things went dark again. The next clear memory I had is waking up in a Colonial Parking Lot kiosk. At some point Helga explained that the guy on the last parking lot shift left the sliding door open and a couple of wool blankets for her every night. It was jarring to wake up next to layers of coats and blankets, hearing babbling nonsense underneath. My entire body was numb. The temperature inside the kiosk had to be hovering around the freezing mark and the odor was foul.

Lying next to Helga, still in my suit and tie, I looked at my watch. It was 7:10 am; I must have slept at least 5 hours. Here I was, new on the job, going out for a couple of drinks after a tough week of work, and waking up next to a bag lady in a parking lot kiosk in my suit. I got up and after sliding the kiosk door, I stepped out and slid the door closed behind me. It was colder, but outside was better than the tiny space inside, all things considered.

With my back to the kiosk, I was having trouble lighting a cigarette. Helga hollered, "Did you break wind in here?"

The noise shot through me; with every cell in my body craving sedation. "No. Absolutely not!"

"Well you certainly stunk up the place. This is my house! Do you understand? My house!"

"Yes. I know it's your place." (I couldn't believe she could smell an additional bad odor because it was fetid to begin with. But I wasn't going to argue with her. I needed a belt of her Kesler's ASAP.)

"Do you know there is blood on your shirt collar?"

I put the tip of my finger on the top of my ear and found fresh blood. Evidently the cut on top of the ear opened up during the night, probably with my tossing and turning. But my immediate concerns were booze for the shakes and finding money to get back to my warm room.

"Are you deaf? I said you have—"

"Yes. I know about the blood. Thanks. I need to figure out how to get home. I have no money. Not even change."

"Where do you live?"

"Langley Park."

Helga slid the door open and stepped out. "You live in a shitty neighborhood. Lots of drugs. Did you know someone was shot and killed trying to buy drugs? A young guy just a few weeks ago. I read it in the Post."

"The Washington Post?" There was probably some incredulity in my voice.

"Why? You don't think some nut like me would read the paper?"

"No. Not at all. I mean of course. I'm not surprised you read the paper. Not at all."

Changing the subject, I asked in a trembling voice, "Do you have any of that whiskey left?"

"Brother you got some nerve. You drank half of my pint last night and now you want the rest? Get lost."

"I just need a sip to calm my jitters."

"Jitters? So, you are an alcoholic. You better check yourself into a treatment program or go to an AA meeting. I can tell you where to go."

I said through chattering teeth, "No thank-you. I simply thought a taste might help warm me up."

"A taste? Sure. I saw how you tasted last night. Go to the AA meeting at St. Mathews Church. It just a few—"

I screamed, "I don't need a fucking AA meeting! I need to calm down and get home!"

"A little sensitive are we fancy pants? Now that's a telltale sign if I ever—"

"Look Helga. I need to get home. I don't know how to get all the way to Langley Park by bus even if I had the money. And let's cut out the bullshit about me being an alcoholic. I'm standing here in my suit!"

Helga looked pensive, finally responding, "Hmmm." Then the agitation came roaring back. "Well that's gratitude for you. And watch your tongue you punk. Don't you get testy with me. I'll fuck you up good!"

As she bent down to pick up her heavy purse, I walked backwards, slowly, about 10 steps. I thanked Helga for the lodging and turned to go, thinking I would have to pan-handle for the change, and I was not going to be shy about asking any drunk I saw for a sip of booze. The anxiety was so intense that I was ready to get physical with a bum if necessary and run away with his bottle or money. I was that desperate.

I only got a few feet when Helga said in a calm voice, a different voice, "Hold on shyster. Here's four dollars in change; that's enough for bus fare and a cup of coffee if you can find one. Walk over to 16th between I and K Streets. There is no J Street in the district. Ask the bus driver where you need to transfer."

When she gave me the money, I promised, "I will find you and pay you back. And I'll give you an extra 20 bucks for a nice meal."

Helga's eyes narrowed and her demeanor changed from kindness to suspicion. She stood there facing me ready to pounce for what seemed like minutes when suddenly she screamed, "You planted something in my brain to read my thoughts. I know who you are. You're a CIA spy. You put a tracking device in my mind."

I turned and began running in a full trot. I looked back several times and saw Helga running after me, but she couldn't keep up. I also reasoned she was not going to leave her cart too far behind, so I slowed to a fast walk on "L" Street going toward 16th Street. Arriving at my destination, I was still out of breath as the bus pulled up. The bus driver gave me a funny look; his eyes went up and down my disheveled suit. I suppose having no coat in such cold added to his curiosity. I mumbled "Fuck him" as I made my way to the back of the empty bus, where I had room to curl up in a fetal position.

My best guess was that Helga was a schizophrenic and was drifting in and out of acute psychosis. Like a lot of homeless people, she was probably off her meds. However, it turned out her instructions were correct; I transferred and the second bus dropped me two blocks from my room.

I wish to parenthetically note that, between the kiosk and blankets, and the money she gave me, there is no question in my mind that Helga saved my life. I remember thinking with the right medication, she might live a relatively normal life.

But the bus ride was a nightmare because I was in acute alcohol withdrawal; I could not stop shaking. I sat rocking back and forth with my hands in my pockets.

At every stop, I almost jumped out thinking I would beg someone for some money to buy a pint. I could think of some pretext and being in a suit might make me more credible. I don't know how I hung on. The feeling is like your mind is going to crack. The fear was that I was going to fall into a psychotic abyss. It is the most extreme kind of anxiety imaginable—an endless panic attack. It would be like a normal person having 100 cups of strong coffee. You will drink anything with alcohol in it—mouthwash or even something dreadful tasting if necessary—to calm down. Only those that have experienced severe alcohol withdrawal know what I'm talking about.

***

I arrived at my apartment building in Langley Park, Maryland, buried in a cluster of two-story buildings, boxes of nondescript fading red brick. As my room key was in my coat that was probably being worn by the mugger, I had to go to the landlady's office to ask her to open the door to my room. If she was not in her office, I was prepared to kick in my door because I needed my credit card to buy booze, but she was there sitting behind her desk. Prudence Higginbottom was a tiny woman, probably in her mid-60s, with light grey hair combed back to a bun. She was the property manager for the entire apartment complex. Prim, brisk, and strict in manner, I never saw her smile. Prudence was another one that gave me a going over that awful morning.

Trying unsuccessfully to hide my tremulousness—it was in my face, hands, and voice—I stammered, "Good morning Miss. Higginbottom. I left my key at work. Could you open my door please?"

After a long, disapproving glare without saying a word, she pulled out an enormous ring with scores of keys out of her desk drawer, rose, and walked out of her office with me close behind. We arrived at my room, but she hesitated, seemingly reluctant to open the door. The landlady turned to me and said, "Do you know you have blood on your shirt?"

"Yes. I had an accident, but I really need to get to bed. It has been a trying morning."

"And no coat. What happened? Did you get mugged?"

"I really don't want to discuss it at this time. If you would just open my door."

I must pause to note that, while it may sound strange, I think it was my suit. If I was in a sweatshirt and blue jeans, I don't think this woman would have given me such a hard time. Nor would the homeless lady think that I was with the CIA. Washington, D.C. has the highest concentration of lawyers in the country. And I believe we are viewed as crooks by the majority. In fact, my sense is that many nonprofessional people have resentments against suits in general. We often (unfairly I contend) represent power, greed, and dishonesty. If you prick us, do we not bleed?

Finally, Miss Higginbottom opened my door. I zipped in while saying thank-you and closed the door. I grabbed my Master Card buried under my socks and underwear and waited a few agonizing minutes to be sure the landlady left the building. When I opened my door, I was shocked to find her still standing there, shaking her head back and forth in disgust.

I blew by the landlady and made a beeline for a bar around the corner. It was 9:50 am, so I had to wait 10 agonizing minutes before the liquor store/bar opened. Tic Toc Liquor Store and Lounge offered no frills—just the promise to be left alone in the dark to get quietly plastered without judgment. It was an oasis of serenity, far from the maddening crowd— the culture wars, ranting of bureaucrats, and the confusing tapestry of regulations. And you could buy a bottle of booze on your way in or out.

Pacing back and forth in front of the liquor store—you had to go through it to get to the bar—I took my pulse. 128 beats per minute; that knowledge sent my heart rate higher. I was still dressed in my rumpled suit. To people passing by, I suppose I looked like a drunk with the shakes, but I didn't give a shit about that. Ditto for the old guy who finally opened the door; I knew that some of his best customers were down and out rummies. I bought a pint of Kessler's whiskey and took two generous slugs. Nerves somewhat steadied, I walked into the bar. Somehow sitting at a bar, even at 10 in the morning, lent some normalcy to my situation. I don't know why that is important but it is. Besides, I had business to attend to: finding my coat, hat, and car keys.

I ordered a bloody Mary and downed it within 30 seconds and ordered another. The bartender's face was in deep shadow—only his big gut barely covered by a thin white dress shirt was visible—but I'm sure he didn't bat an eyelash. There was nothing special about Tic Tock's Bloody Mary's: a shot of vodka in some cheap tomato juice. Forget about a stalk of celery or Worcestershire sauce. After the Kesler's and a second Bloody Mary that I was able to sip, I was sufficiently calm to go over what I remembered. I called the Fox from a public phone on the wall, which is a unique feature of the Toc. I didn't expect anyone to answer so early in the day, but some grumpy guy did. I asked about my coat.

"Can you describe it?"

"Yes. It is black wool with a Brook's Brothers label. There is a New Orleans Saints ring with four keys on it. I think my coat is on a hook near the door."

During a period of silence, still thinking it was more likely that the mugger got my coat, I prayed to St. Anthony, the patron saint of lost things. Within a few seconds of that prayer I heard, "Yeah. It's here buddy."

"Are the keys in the coat?"

"The keys are in the coat. So are an egg roll and a piece of pizza that I got all over my hand."

"Sorry about that. Is there a hat?"

"No hat. We open at 2 pm. Next time call after 2." Click.

I thought how utterly odd. Why didn't I eat those appetizers at the Fox? Maybe I took them to go and changed my mind about leaving. My fedora could have ended up in any number of bars or with the mugger, but I had lost many hats; it was part of the price one pays to have a good time. Moreover, with coat and keys secured, I was overflowing with gratitude. With that worry out of the way, I sat at the bar, ordered another drink, thanked Saint Anthony, let out a long sigh of relief, and whispered, "I survived that fiasco relatively unscathed."

A guy came into the Toc and sat two stools from me. I couldn't see him well, but I knew it was Fred from his wheezing and disgusting, rattling cough. I told Fred about what had happened. I added, "I guess the fact that I could so easily dismiss what had transpired the previous 12 hours; that is, carry on as if nothing happened is not normal."

Leaning over and looking into his drink—I could see Fred's large profile in deep shadow—he sardonically answered, "That is definitely not normal Ralph. None of it. I think you should seriously think about seeing a psychiatrist."

I considered the source for that malicious remark; unlike a guy like me who frequented high end cocktail lounges with music and beautiful women, Fred was a lush and only drank at the Toc and a few other shit-holes in the neighborhood by himself.

***

I managed to pull myself out of the bar while still ambulatory, took the bus in a relaxed manner, retrieved my coat, and picked up my car. I came back to my room and polished off what was left of the whiskey. I sweated out Sunday tapering off with beer. But I was profoundly grateful to be back in my room, safe and warm, sitting up in my bed against several pillows, watching re-runs of The Love Boat and Fantasy Island on my small black and white TV with a coat hanger for an antenna.

Upon awakening Monday morning, I was immediately greeted by intense fear of someone from work seeing me with the homeless woman, even knowing that the odds of such a thing were astronomical. The fear may sound irrational, but I knew co-workers who went out after work and Pennsylvania Avenue is a main thoroughfare. Anybody living in Virginia would probably use it and most of them did live across the Potomac River. I was creating this horrific scenario with dialogue in my head. "Hey, isn't that the new guy Rogers with a bag lady." There was no mistaking who she was wearing a loud overcoat, pushing an overflowing shopping cart. They would end up thinking I was with her to have sex. "Hey, that new guy Rogers must be some kind of a freak!"

I cried out, "Dear God in heaven, my reputation will be destroyed. I just got here!" That paranoia persisted for months.

I did make a good faith effort to find Helga. To be honest, I was somewhat relieved in not seeing her on K Street. I didn't care about the twenty-four bucks. I obviously could have gone to the parking lot kiosk, but that meant either 3 am or upon sunrise, and I was not going to run the risk of being exposed again. I also didn't pray to St. Anthony for help in finding Helga on K Street, but I don't feel guilty about that. I don't even believe in God let alone some saint that finds lost stuff for you.

***

More than a year later, when the spring weather arrived, I began taking a longer walk from the Farragut Square metro stop to my job for the exercise. I passed a well-dressed woman, calmly sitting on a bench in Lafayette Park with her legs crossed. She had a snub nose and attractive silver white hair draping her ears and forehead. The woman could not have more than 60, and her clothes were stunning: a wide brimmed, turquoise hat; a pleated turquoise skirt; a chic black blouse; and black heels. My roving eyes returned to the small nose, but I laughed at the thought that it could be Helga. She looked more like the lovely British actress Dame Helen Mirren only better dressed.

The woman followed me with her eyes as I walked by. She did not move a muscle. When I looked back, her head had turned and she was still staring at me without expression. It was eerie.

The next morning, the stylish mystery woman was on the same bench, dressed in yellow and black, including a wide-brimmed black hat, what looked like long, black silk gloves; and large, round sunglasses. Her attire reminded me of an older Audrey Hepburn's Highly-go-Lightly. A long cigarette holder would not have looked out of place. I wanted to stop and speak to her, but I was quite nervous that morning. I drank a lot the night before during a rare work-night out. That was happening more frequently I have to admit. Instead, I stopped a few benches away, sat down, pulled out a pint of vodka from inside my briefcase, and took a couple of gulps to calm down. The lady's head was turned toward me and she had a wry smile. I had never seen a woman dressed so fashionable, not in lackluster Washington, D.C. anyway.

I was surprised at the degree of withdrawal after only one night out. I made it to work and stayed put, with the help of what was left of the pint of booze, but I had to replace it by lunch-time. While on the job, it was always a delicate balance between taking the edge off and slipping into visible intoxication with a staggering drunk not far behind, without a clue as to how grossly intoxicated I appeared to others. Moreover, while the barroom atmosphere is always a big part of the attraction for me; drinking in bathroom stalls is not.

That night, sitting in my bed propped up by several pillows, I thought about the woman in the park. As I took only small sips of Kesler's whiskey, I reasoned the only way it could have been Helga is if she had had Botox injections to remove all the facial wrinkles and dermabrasion to have such clear skin. And perhaps a face lift as she somehow got rid of that prominent chin. I laughed at my absurd analysis, although Betty Davis in the movie "Pocketful Of Miracles" occurred to me; she went from a bag lady to a stunning mother comfortable to meet her daughter and her fiancé, a Spanish prince. While thinking it was ridiculous applying the premise of the movie to the fashionable lady in the park, the snub nose and unnatural lengthy stare gave me pause that evening.

On the third day, I was still a bit jittery from the last drunk, or maybe the well-dressed woman unnerved me, but rather than taking a different route, I felt compelled to see if she was in the park again. A light rain was falling as I entered Lafayette Park directly in front of the white house. No more than 50 yards away, the same woman, dressed in black with fuchsia-colored heels with a matching umbrella, stood up from a bench and walked in the opposite direction from where I was standing. I could have caught up to her, but it began raining hard and I forgot my umbrella. She stopped, turned back, and smiled under her umbrella. As she continued on through the park, I noticed a pronounced limp on the right.

***

Was I hallucinating? Possibly; in retrospect, my alcoholism, including more frequent visual hallucinations, was progressing as it always does. But essentially the same illusion on three consecutive days? The snub nose and the starring and the limp on the right; the weight of the evidence supported this conclusion: it was Helga, stabilized on anti-psychotic medication, followed by a total make-over, going from rags to riches.

I was fired within six months of seeing Helga in the park, for being grossly intoxicated during working hours and hovering over a co-worker's desk, with alcohol breath, saying she was the most beautiful women in the Department of Justice.

My drinking increased. I'm in a D.C. men's shelter as I write, trying to put the plug in the jug and figuring out my next move. What a reversal of fortune: from the bag lady and the suit to the belle and the bum.

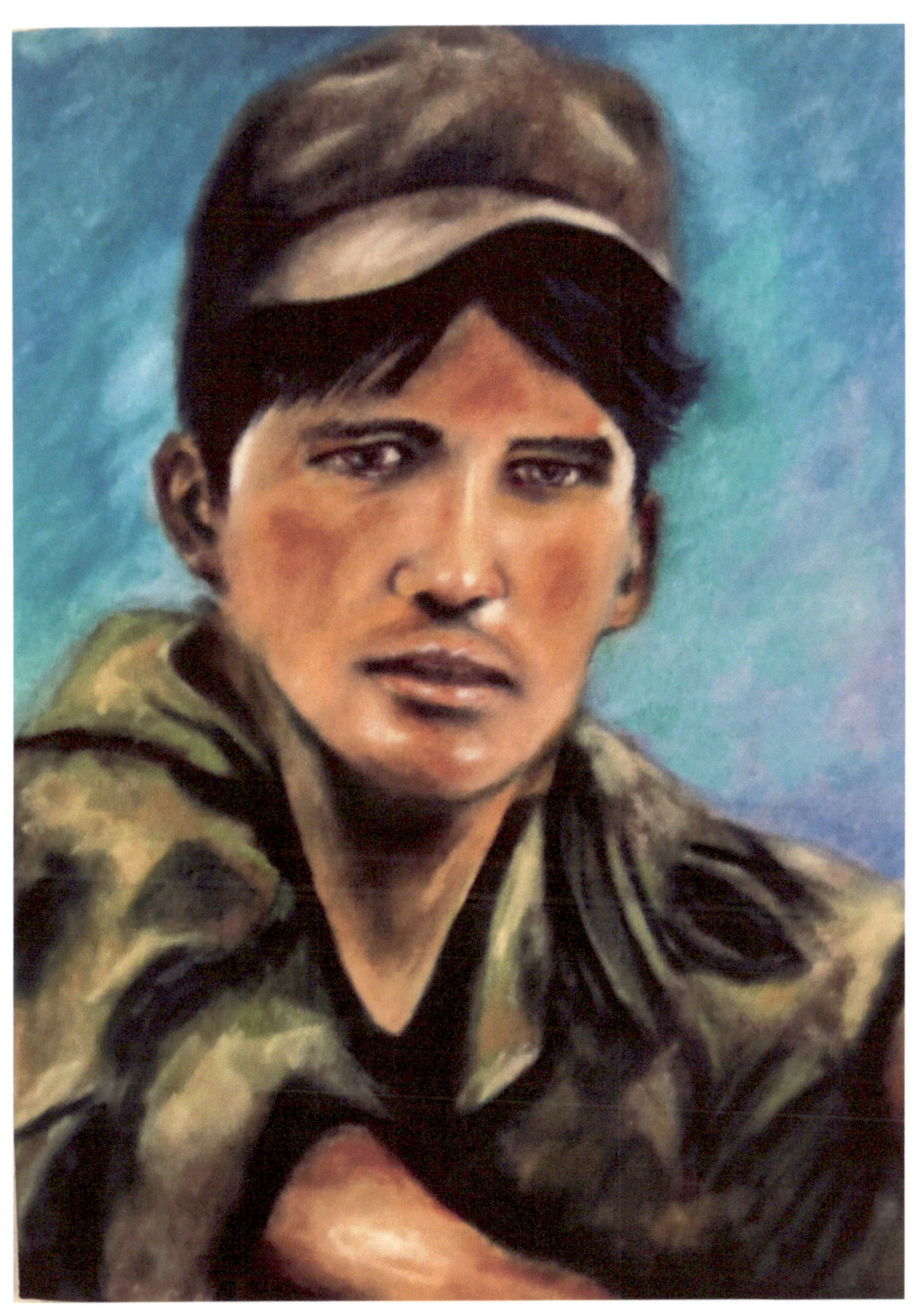

Tom Mulligan
Vietnam
Private Collection

The Big Jig Was Up

I suddenly awoke in a panic, sweating profusely. Every cell in my body was in a state of agitation as my blood alcohol level was falling precipitously. My first coherent thought was that I did not have any booze or sedative to calm my shakes, which triggered a more intense wave of panic. As I lay in bed clutching a pillow and closing my eyes to a blinding white light on the ceiling left on by my wife, in disbelief that I did not plan ahead to have my usual pint of vodka within reach, I was going to unclench and scream for an immediate and sufficient amount of alcohol to prevent potentially lethal DT's, my secret be damned. My mother and wife certainly suspected I had a drinking problem and that was all right. But the alcoholic is at his most vulnerable in acute withdrawal; let them see the embarrassing and bizarre behavior and I won't try and deny blackouts, but I'd rather slit my throat than have a loved one seeing a pitiful shaking drunk gulping booze at 8 am. Yet here I was with no alternative but to bare my shuddering soul.

By what I considered at the time to be divine intervention, a memory broke through a tangled web of misfiring neurons: a nearly full liter of Canadian Club whiskey that my mother kept for medicinal purposes—it went down about a shot a year and I never had need to disturb it—was sitting pretty in her hallway closet. I had an urgent need for my medication: two generous belts to stave of DTs. Thereafter, I could put the next shot in my coffee and mingle with family on that Christmas morning, admiring the perfectly shaped and adorned tree with the delightful smell of pine, looking perfectly jolly, which always pleases my mother. She is enamored to my alcoholic personality and why not? I am not a disagreeable drunk. On the contrary, I converse affably, smile, and occasionally laugh. I'm a boring stiff sober.

Without saying a word to my wife sitting quietly at the kitchen table reading the morning paper, or my mother scurrying about with the clanging of pots and pans, I quietly opened the closet door with a laughing red Santa towel in hand so that I could slide the bottle of whiskey out without detection, but I was stunned to find the fifth was gone. I silently shrieked at a terror-filled image of cracks in my brain that would soon shatter like glass into countless, useless pieces.

In bright red robe and red slippers, I was vibrating in place, ready to cry out for help, divulging an awful truth that by itself is diagnostic of alcoholism, when a sudden thought burst forth giving me a momentary respite—no, it was more akin to a slight decrease in panic. Showered by Grace, the face-saving, perhaps lifesaving memory was there are a bunch of 16 once beers in the fridge.

I nodded good morning to my wife and mother without making eye contact, mumbled something about coffee cream and stealthily slipped one can of beer in each pocket of my robe behind the refrigerator door. With liquor, sufficient sedation was instantaneous and it rarely caused vomiting. I can't stand chugging beer under such circumstances; it always makes me want to puke. But I had no choice; the beer would have to suffice.

I tip-toed out of view with a plan to drink the beers in the bathroom, but my hung-over cousin Tom was locked in; with my ear pressed to the door, I only heard a series of alternating wheezing and gurgling noises, followed by a long death-like moan. I had a fleeting realization of where the Canadian Club whiskey went—my cousin is a lying, thieving lush— but I had a much more pressing issue to attend to.

In the meantime, my wife Niki went back to the bedroom we were using; she was lying down with a wet, green washcloth over her forehead and eyes and mumbled something about not being able to stand it any more. I'm not sure if she was referring to me or my mother. My stepfather Winthrop, whose bowed face was covered by long stringy grey hair, sat on the edge of his bed in the other bedroom, transfixed by what was on a calculator in his hand, solving complex calculus problems, no doubt. What a weird fuck that guy is.

Thwarted at every turn, perspiring profusely and visibly shaking, I put my camel hair coat over my robe, grabbed two more 16 once beers out of the fridge, stuck them into my outer pockets without being detected, and said to my mother while on the move that I had to go to my car to find some work-related papers. She must have been aware of the winter storm outside but, red-faced and perspiring from all that was in and on the stove, she did not notice that her son was still in his slippers.

Holding on for dear life and despite being caught in the terrifying vise of severe withdrawal necessitating instant sedation and desperately trying to avoid being detected in how I had to relieve such a state, I had the presence of mind to come up with such a credible pretext: work-related papers in my car. (Being safely removed from the horror in time and space, I can appreciate the beauty of it; drinking in peace and if subsequently challenged on the amount of time it took, I could explain that I had to go through all of the papers to make sure I had the right material.) Besides, my mother was an easy mark. My wife was another story. Credible lies can be more intuitive than conscious with the alcoholic. But at this stage of my marriage to Niki, there was a certain amount of suspicion no matter what I was up to. I was treading on thin ice.

I went out of the house and walked briskly through a blinding blizzard, my overcoat billowing in the icy breeze with only thin red PJs underneath. I was literally freezing my ass off, but that was not my primary concern. I knew that with a history of hallucinations and two seizures, the escalating withdrawal was life-threatening. I found rows of snow-covered cars in both directions. I suspected Niki drove us home, but I had no memory of where the car was parked. The last few hours of the previous night were blank.

Wildly brushing cars like Jack Lemon with the flower pots, hands red and raw, I found and entered my car. My feet and ankles were bone cracking cold after walking through 6 inches of fresh snow. With my car frigid but running, I got the first 16 once beer down, gagging but mercifully not vomiting. However, 16 ounces of 4.6% beer was not nearly enough alcohol to take the edge off. Looking through the frost-covered windshield at the back of a huge plow pushing the snow to its left, leaving an impenetrable wall to my right, the second can of beer was not going down too well either. I needed a minimum of 48 ounces to calm down and give me time to figure out my next move.

As the third can of beer was an inch from my lips, held in suspension while retching, I noticed a dark, blurry figure moving quickly through a blowing white sheath, coming toward me. Within a few seconds, a gloved hand was brushing off the snow on my side window. It was Niki with bulging eyes and an open mouth like the raging head of Medusa. After looking at the 16 once beer can in my hand, her eyes moved to the soaking wet slippers on my feet. I was frozen in fear. What could I say? "I know it's a bit early honey, but I felt like having a beer in my car." The jig was up.

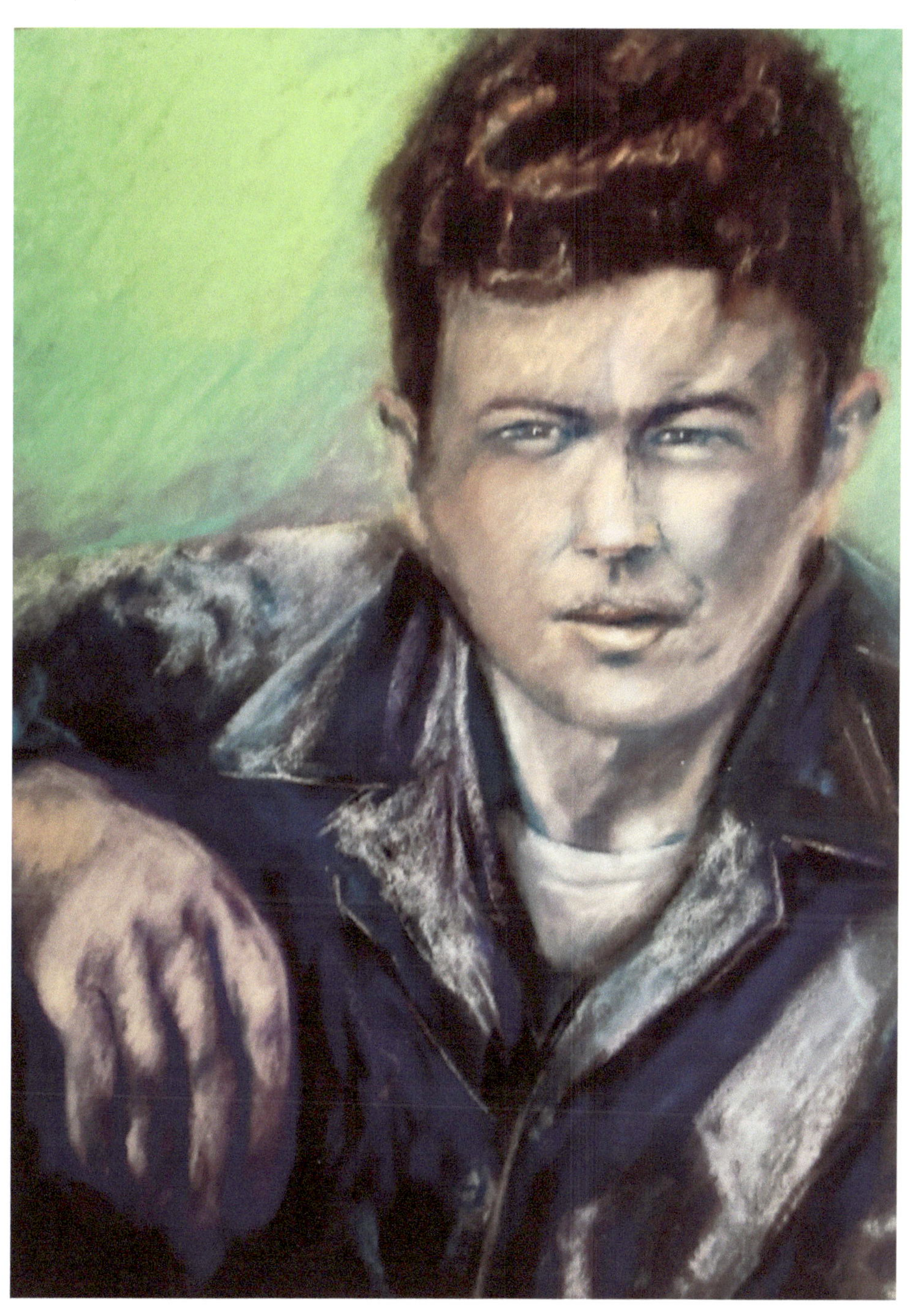

James Mulligan, Age 26
KIA, WW II
Bougainville

Connie Salvatore

Wearing a white First Communion dress, Connie was holding her mother's hand, in front of their small red brick house, waiting by the curb. Connie was smiling and laughed when she looked up at her mother. I would eventually learn that was her normal disposition—the polar opposite of me—that was part of her charm.

The Salvatore family lived on Cottage Street, just one block from my house on Allen. Connie could have been mistaken for a Filipina, although that is with knowledge I have today; I could not have known such an ethnicity back then. My world was very small; I was only 9 years old, a year older than Connie. I was simply drawn to her large eyes; they were of a different shape from all the other girls, mesmeric in their beauty.

It was not love—to call it that at such a young age would be absurd—but it was a very strong infatuation at first sight. I was standing on the other side of the street staring, immobilized by awe. She looked at me curiously—a do I know this boy look—but I don't think I registered in her conscious. That is, whatever thought she had while looking at me was gone the moment her eyes went elsewhere. I believe the feeling I had was for her beauty—nothing more than that—but it was honest and pure. I have deep sorrow for never telling her that.

Connie had straight black hair, cut leaving bangs over her forehead to her eyebrows, and the rest of the hair was slightly longer all the way around; it was a cute little girl's bowl cut. I experienced a longing because of her eyes and straight hair that was the blackest black I had ever seen. I could not reveal myself—a sliver of a blonde boy who blushed upon a glance—therefore, I had to gaze upon her from a distance or day dream.

I remember putting a transistor radio under my pillow at night and every time I heard a song about wanting or loving a girl, I thought about Connie. I fantasized about the two of us being together. There was nothing sexual about it; I knew nothing about that at age 9. I only wanted to be with her, with her acknowledging me, wanting to be with me, and that was as sincere a feeling as I have ever had.

Forty-six years later, in April 2003, profoundly depressed despite being on anti-depressant medication for close to a year, and still contemplating suicide, I decided to see a therapist. Dr. Judith Shapiro, a psychologist, who had an office in her home in Amherst, a wealthy Buffalo, New York suburb. The sky was growing darker and I heard several claps of thunder as I walked up the long driveway that curved left and up. While looking at a three-story white Victorian home with steeply pitched roofs of irregular shapes, towers, and turrets, and many overhangs with windows, it looked like a foreboding castle. Dr. Shapiro answered the door and escorted me to her office in the furnished basement. There were several bookcases filled with volumes on psychology and sociology, among other things. The office was dimly lit with a white shag carpet and white leather couch with large black cushions. The psychologist was short in stature, 50ish, plump, with thick glasses. She had short, straight grey hair. Business-like in manner and pleasant, there was also a bumbling way about her that I found easy to connect with.

After the usual introductory information and giving the psychologist my childhood memories of Connie, Dr. Shapiro, sitting in a white leather chair to the right of her desk and directly across from me, pulled her charcoal grey skirt well below her knees, and pushing herself up with the palms of her hands to readjust her sitting position—a ritual she would repeat every few minutes—asked, "Did you ever see her again?"

"Yes. I saw her many times as a teenager in high school; she was always walking with 2 or 3 girls, carrying her books close to her chest, with me gazing from a distance. She was beautiful with the same gorgeous eyes. And as is typical with good-looking girls, she knew how to dress: stylishly and sexy but not overdoing it. I remember in particular tight blue jeans with a crisp white blouse and high collar that looked stunning next to her olive skin tone and black hair. She wore cashmere sweaters of black and red and pink, and I was of an age to be attracted to her sensual body.

"With her captivating personality, photogenic smile—she never wore a frown—she was absolute perfection. Connie's looks, personality, laugh, the way she talked, her mannerisms—I would not have changed one thing about her. I was in one of her classes; typing was an elective course that I had no interest in, so I saw her up close 5 days a week without opening my mouth. I trembled upon a mere glimpse from her.

"Aside from the shyness, by the time I was a junior at Lafayette High School, I saw myself as way out of her league and was afraid of rejection. But at the end of my junior year, after a six-pack of beer, I stood in the back of a delicatessen and called her using a public wall phone and asked her to my high school ring dance, which was like a prom but for juniors. I was pleasantly surprised when she said yes. Actually, I was flabbergasted.

"There must have been a hundred of us that went to a fancy restaurant with white linen and wine glasses and waiters in tuxedos. I slow danced with Connie to the tune of "I Only Have Eyes For You" by the Flamingos and for a moment, gazed into her green eyes. I have never felt that degree of warmth, tenderness, and adoration again.

"Unfortunately, at 17, being immature and not knowing how to act in such a place with a pretty girl, I drank too much with a fake ID. I was with the girl of my dreams, never expecting I would have such an opportunity, and I blew it. We took a cab with another couple. I was in a blackout by then and didn't even walk Connie to her door. I know that because she told me the next time I saw her, weeks after the dance. She was on the other side of the street with girlfriends and shouted it at me from a distance.

"I could have called her up and apologized, asked her for another chance—something; anything—I can't explain why I just dropped it. It wasn't just my actions; it's difficult to fathom what was left unsaid."

"Did you ever see Connie after that?"

"Twice. I was living in a cottage on the lake with 8 other guys during the summer of 1970. We called it "Cold Duck", which gives you an idea of what we were about that summer."

"I don't follow?"

"Cold Duck. Cheap wine. We had a painting of a bottle of it on the front of our cottage, above the door."

"Oh."

(I could tell the psychologist did not know anything about cheap wine.)

"Most of us weren't working as we just came out of the service, four of us from Vietnam. We drank every day. Not just cheap wine; beer trucks delivered many cases of Genesee beer every week. It was like Animal House."

"I see."

(She had no idea what I was talking about.)

"Connie and a couple of her girlfriends visited our cottage. I think they were merely making the rounds, going from cottage to cottage as there were many of them filled with young people having parties. On this particular night, I had a garbage can over my head—an empty one—that had a rust hole where my eyes were so I recognized Connie and said hi. She must have recognized my voice or maybe my eyes through the hole because she said in a sad voice, "Oh Louis." Maybe she was disappointed that I would walk around like that. I was always looking for a laugh. Some laugh."

Dr. Shapiro leaned forward with expanding eyes and observed, "You literally put your head in a garbage can. Fascinating."

Sitting up straight on the edge of the couch, I said with sadness, "The thing that made a relationship impossible was my shyness."

"And getting plastered with a garbage can over your head."

I answered, "That too."

Dr. Shapiro wrote something on her pad while asking, "Was Connie oriental?"

"No. She was Italian. Connie Salvatore."

"Interesting. Did you know that Salvatore means savior in Italian?"

"It does? Well, I have been looking to be saved from as far back as I can remember; to be pulled out of the depths of despair. But it was more than that; I have been chasing after that magical feeling I had for Connie all these years and I've never found it."

"Feeling?"

"When I had her in my arms and looked into her eyes. It was merely seconds but there's not a day that has gone by that I haven't thought about how I felt in that moment. The first feelings of passion wrapped in idyllic love can be quite powerful I guess."

Dr. Shapiro looked past me and sighed, "It can indeed."

I turned my head and looked out a window; it was windy and raining hard with several bamboo trees swaying violently in the wind. Still looking out the window, I wondered out loud, "There was such purity about it; totally innocent; a longing with no hidden agenda. It was beautiful. And she did come to my cottage. Maybe she came to see me."

I turned to Dr. Shapiro and asked, "Why didn't I ever consider that? I never followed up with anything. Not even a phone call. I can't explain that."

"That's why you are here Louis. You said you saw Connie again twice. When did you see her the last time?"

"A week ago, more than thirty years after that unfortunate encounter with the garbage can. I just turned 52, which makes her 51."

There was an uncomfortable pause waiting for the next question.

Dr. Shapiro raised her eyebrows and with a rising voice asked, "And?"

"I heard it through the grapevine that Connie was divorced and living alone in West Palm Beach, Florida. I had just come out of a painful divorce myself."

Dr. Shapiro asked, "Did you go to Florida to see her?"

"Do you mind if I stand?"

"Not at all Louis."

I stood up and walked to the small open window to the large back yard.

I could hear the wind howling and the bamboo trees were bent so far that they were U-shaped. The rain had stopped. I deeply inhaled the pleasant smell of freshly cut grass and rain. There were three small cherry trees with pinkish-white blossoms scattered all over the lawn. Many blossoms were floating, swirling, before they gently touched down.

I turned to the psychologist and finally answered, "Yes. I went to see her unannounced. I knew it could blow up in my face. She might be living with a guy or upset at me showing up out of the blue. Or worse; I might have been only a blip at best on her romantic screen with her looking at me incredulous. But there was no choice in the matter. The fantasy was like a drug; it was sometimes lovely but more often painful. It hurt because I missed my chance and had a string of broken relationships thereafter. I lived with a woman I did not love for 15 years. But I barely knew Connie; maybe it was about something else?"

Dr. Shapiro interjected, "It could very well be. We will eventually take a look at that. But please continue Louis."

"I had her address and phone number from a friend of a friend. Notwithstanding the third hand information of an unknown age, I flew to Miami and rented a powder blue Mustang convertible from the airport that I had reserved. I thought of everything and was going to pull out all the stops. Dressed in blue jeans; black elk skin, pointed cowboy boots; a fuchsia polo shirt; a fuchsia suitcoat with black kerchief; and a black felt hat with a short brim, I wondered if my attire was a bit much, but I dismissed that concern as my destination was Palm Beach and Connie and why not show up as me.

"It was sunny and balmy with a slight breeze. Driving up I-95 for two hours with the top down, I was able to find the house in West Palm with my GPS. I was surprised by the neighborhood; most of the houses were small wooden structures, but they were maintained well with manicured lawns.

"I found Connie's small house on Everglade Lane, a narrow street that sloped downward. I parked in front and looked at the box-like structure painted white with blue trim, but it was badly in need of fresh paint as it was bubbling up and peeling on each side of the front door and above the large picture window. There were two palm trees that framed the house, with many twisted brown-colored leaves hanging by a thread or lying curled up and dead on the ground. The grass on the lawn was high and fading green bushes in front of the house were being strangled by long, spiny weeds. I walked on the walkway to the door; there were many broken and missing pieces of cement with one sharp piece jutting out just before the stoop in front of the door. Hyperventilating and light-headed, I stood at the door trying to compose myself.”

Dr. Shapiro leaned forward and looked captivated by my story; she let me continue without making a remark.

“I rang the doorbell twice but after no response, I opened the screen door and knocked on the wooden door. I waited a minute and knocked again very hard. I didn’t hear a sound and there was no car in the driveway. I waited for a couple of minutes after knocking a third time. As I walked toward my car, I heard a creaking sound. I turned and walked back while looking at an old man, pale-faced and bald with a long unkempt white beard that reached his mid-chest. As I drew near, he squinted at me through the screen door.

“Hunched over, wearing a red plaid shirt with blue-jean overhauls and straps over his shoulders, he reeked of whiskey.

“I asked if Connie Salvatore lived there.

“In a raspy voice through labored breathing, he answered, ‘Connie who?’

“Connie Salvatore.”

“The old man pulled on his beard and said, ‘No. But there’s a Connie Barone here.’

“I answered, ‘It must be her.’

“The old man opened the door and pointed to a couch and said, ‘Come in and have a seat.’

“Slightly bent over, he shuffled through the living room and turned a corner into a dark hall. I was surprised the old man didn’t ask my name, but I was glad he didn’t. I wanted to meet Connie without notice, suddenly, and concentrate on what her eyes told me.”

“I stood in the foyer and looked into the living room. The only furniture consisted of a dark wood coffee table, two large chairs, and the couch, all upholstered grey and thread bare. I sat on the edge of the middle of the couch. There was a strong musty smell. Looking about the room, I saw nothing on the greying white walls. Feeling excitement mixed with bewilderment and fear, I sneezed several times from the dust visibly floating inside a ray of light coming through a narrow opening of the middle of the curtains in the front window.

“There was a framed photo of a young girl on the mantle above a fireplace; she was dressed in a blue and green plaid skirt with blue straps over a white blouse, had a black hair bowl cut with bangs covering her forehead, and beguiling eyes. An identical photo was in a silver frame on the glass coffee table in front of the couch. The little girl was Connie. Looking back and forth, I wondered why anyone would have the same two photos and nothing else in a living room, but I was too excited to dwell on anything other than Connie in her pink strapless prom dress, black hair, and big green eyes. I became distracted by a spider slowly moving toward a struggling fly trapped in a web connecting the framed photo on the mantle to the wall.

"Disjointed thoughts and emotions swept through me in waves. I thought the old man must be a relative, how would she receive me—she might be upset or worse not remember me—and wondered what she looked like. I knew at a minimum I would see her. Looking at the photo nearest me, I was hoping to take her out for dinner and tell her how I felt about her when we were young. I fantasized about dancing with her like we did decades ago. But my mind couldn't stay with that lovely vision; rather, it jumped from how could the old guy be her mate to probably he was a boarder to possibly he was her father to maybe she saw me out front and is taking time getting ready to her awkwardly asking, 'Why are you here?'

"I looked at the dark entrance to the hallway and back to the photo of the Connie of my childhood. Thinking of the reservations I made at Swifty's, an elegant restaurant at the Colony Hotel in Palm Beach, I thought it was possible she would appreciate my hutzpah and holding on to this romantic dream for so many years. But that thought was quickly supplanted by Jay Gatsby returning to Daisey after only a few years and look how that turned out. Here was I decades later after a dance. I came a long way from a long time ago, bursting forth like a clownish jack-in-the-box."

Dr. Shapiro interjected, "This is quite a story Louis. Do you want to pause and consider what you have said thus far?"

I answered, "No. Please. Let me continue. I'm almost done."

"O.K. That's fine."

I stood up and walked over to the window again. It was still windy and all the pinkish-white blossoms were no longer on the grass. I turned and looked at the psychologist. "As an old woman with a black cane slowly walked into the living room and approached me, I stood up and assumed she was the old man's wife. She was short, slightly hunched over, with thinning grey hair covered by a yellow scarf. She had spider wrinkles that spun in all directions from her eyes and mouth; a thick, quivering lower lip; and deep crevices in both cheeks. Was she Connie's mother? The old man said Connie Barone. It occurred to me that Italian mothers and daughters sometimes have the same first name. Fidgety, pulling the edges of my suitcoat down and scratching my nose, I was squirming in my sweating skin.

"She glared at me for a few seconds as I looked into her sunken eyes.

They were a pale green, with a long distance between the eyebrow and eyelash. I felt a mixture of shock and sadness.

"With sudden slits for eyes, she asked, 'Who are you?'

"I stammered my name; mentioned the ring dance; the names of the streets from our childhood; and while out of breath, the names of some mutual friends from our teenage years. I felt heat on my face and my throat was very dry.

"As she pointed her black cane at me and scowled, her body stiffened like a cat ready to pounce. She hissed, 'How did you get my address?'

"I answered, 'I asked around the old neighborhood. I hope you—'

"With a low voice like she was possessed, she howled, 'I have no idea what you're up to, but you better get the hell out of my house and off of my property or I'll call the police.'

"I shivered and mumbled an apology on my way to the door, stopped, turned to face her, and pleaded, 'Do you remember me?'

"Connie raised her cane and pushed the end of it into my chest. I turned and opened the screen door and stepped out, but I stopped and turned around to look at her again and implored, 'Connie'

"She took two steps forward and pushed the wooden door shut.

"I was stunned. With my head hanging down, I stumbled over the broken cement walkway to my car. With my right hand above the car door for support, I turned to look at the picture window on the front of the house and noticed a hand holding the edge of a white curtain open. I saw the yellow scarf over a gaunt face. We looked at each other for what seemed like several minutes until the curtain closed."

✳✳✳

After a few moments of silence, the psychologist said, "I'm so sorry Louis. How disappointing to find Connie in such a state."

"I don't believe it was Connie."

"What?"

"I initially thought it was and was devastated. I drove to the Colony, walked into the dining room, and was ushered to my reserved table while lying that I was waiting for my wife. But as I looked around the room seeing so many happy couples, it was too depressing. I got up and without saying a word to anyone, walked outside to a bar by a pool close to the beach. It was dusk and clouds were tinged with fading oranges and reds that soon gave way to pale pinks and dark purples and darkness. Glowing Tiki lamps were scattered around the bar and white tables. There were 4 or 5 empty stools at the small bar manned by a young man with bleach-blonde hair, dressed in white shorts and an open white shirt, with a bronze tan and brilliant white teeth. I sat and ordered a gin and tonic. I gulped it down and ordered another. I was literally swallowing bitter anguish after having planned this affair for years. I watched the waves crashing onto the beach below. There was stiff breeze that blew my cocktail napkin off the bar.

"I swung around on the stool to look at the people sitting at the half a dozen tables under several clusters of palm trees. Some faces were in dark shadow but others were illuminated by the Tiki lamps. I was suddenly struck by two women laughing; they were facing me, no more than 30 yards away. I believe one of the women was Connie. Remarkably, she had the same face and eyes; the same body from what I could tell."

Dr, Shapiro uttered an unprofessional, "Wow! Are you sure?"

I answered, "Yes. In addition to the physical characteristics, she had the same laugh. I heard her distinct laugh; it was more like a giggle. And she looked at me curiously, exactly like she did when we were children. It was this I think I know this guy kind of look, but she resumed her conversation with her friend followed by a giggle. I was in and out of her consciousnesses within a few seconds, confirming what I feared."

"Confirming what Louis?"

"That I never mattered to her. Here I have been fantasizing about Connie all these years and she takes one look at me— I was invalidated; dismissed as unworthy of anything more than a moment of reflection.

"I put two 20-dollar bills on the bar, got up and with legs like rubber, walked through the hotel to the parking valet. After shaking and sobbing in the car for a long time, I drove back to Miami."

"After such an ordeal to see her, why didn't you at least introduce yourself? Isn't it possible you read Connie's look wrong? That maybe she didn't recognize you?"

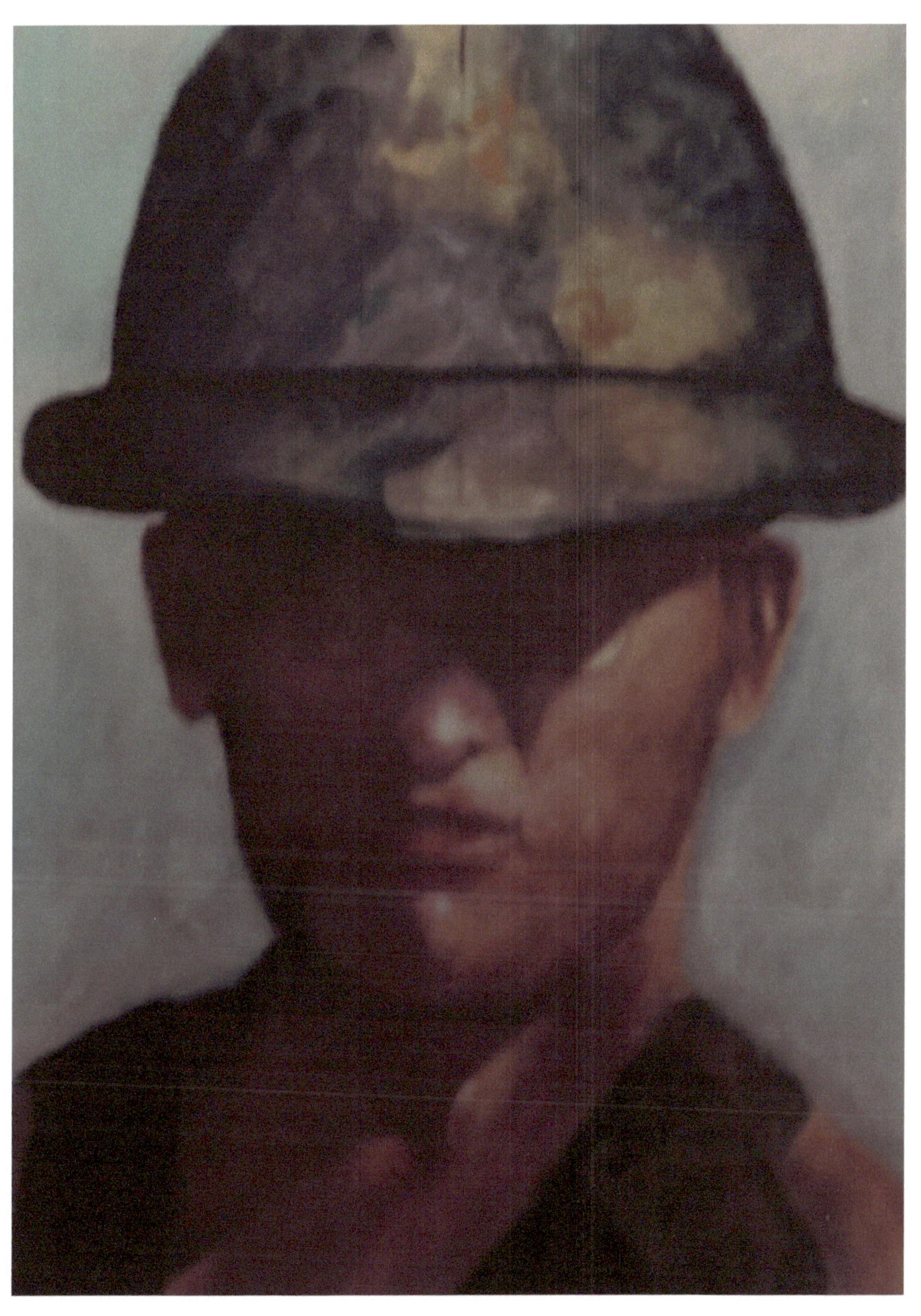

Carl, Age 22
Vietnam, KIA
Buffalo VA Regional Office

A Cunning and Baffling Progressive Disease

***

Freddie and Oscar: Round One

My wife called me a booze hound with denial, rationalization, and a mental obsession, staggering toward a catastrophe. I thought her uneducated opinion on the matter was wildly off the mark, but she had leverage and lowered the boom. Walking up a winding sidewalk to a two-story red brick building, I felt indignant about being forced to take off from work to talk with a stranger about my drinking. I was further incensed when no one responded to my knocks on a locked front door, nor to pounding on a locked side door. I yelled, "What kind of bullshit is this? Are you locking people in or out?"

I paid no attention to a pile of blankets to my left until a face full of hair popped up yelling, "What the fuck do you want?" After informing this nut case of my intention, he howled, "It's on the other side." A drunken bum who stunk to the high heavens on the doorstep; needless to say, I was not impressed with the Easy Does It alcohol and drug rehabilitation program thus far. After finally finding one of multiple rear doors open, my long walk down a corridor changed my sour mood to fear; it felt like I had been summoned to the principal's office.

Looking at my scribble of a number on a piece of paper, I found the right office, saw a blurred, seated image through the frosted glass, and gently knocked. A loud, "Come in" shot through me. I inexplicably didn't steady my nerves in the car as vodka doesn't smell. Oscar Stanley Fuentes rose as I entered the room. He was only about 5 foot 6 inches, but his tight black polo shirt enhanced bulging muscles that I would eventually learn were from daily work-outs with weights that began during a 5-year stint at Attica for doing something bad that he didn't remember doing. I was initially intimidated by his clean-shaven head and strange animal tattoos up and down his arms. His flat affect and interrogating eyes were also disquieting. A gold ring earring made him look like a mean Mr. Clean.

With arched eyebrows, Yul Byrnner also came to mind. Standing in front of his desk, it felt like the judge had already reached his verdict.

Tall and thin with neatly cut black hair parted on the right, I was wearing a dark blue pinstripe suit, light blue shirt, yellow tie, and tinted glasses. I thought it was important to make a good impression, and I hasten to add the accurate one. I was not some alky out in the street hovering in a doorway with a liter of cheap booze in a brown paper bag.

After introducing himself in a deep, gravelly voice, Oscar asked me to sit in an uncomfortable wooden chair in front of his desk. No wonder I felt intimidated now that I remember this set up; I had pictured a soft leather couch with pillows. Oscar was in a dark green chair with a lot of padding. We sat facing each other.

With his right index and forefingers, Oscar pushed his black framed glasses on top of his bald head and said, "Good morning Mr. Baumgarten. My name is Oscar Fuentes. I am a certified alcohol and drug counselor with Easy Does It. May I call you Fred?"

"Freddie."

"OK Freddie. Please call me Oscar. I am a recovering alcoholic and drug addict with 19 years of sobriety, and I've been a counselor with Easy Does It for the past 12 years. (I thought, big fucking deal.) I would like to get right to the point. Do you think you are an alcoholic?"

"Technically yes, but with an asterisk."

With furrowed brow, Oscar inquired, "Why the asterisk?"

"I believe I'm a functional alcoholic. I do have blackouts and morning shakes, but I have never been a daily drinker, nor have I lost a job. I began having alcohol withdrawal symptoms in my mid-20s. That culminated in an episode of delirium tremens in my early 30s while, fortunately, hospitalized for alcohol detoxification. For most of my drinking career, that has been the culprit right there."

With black bushy eyebrows raised, Oscar queried, "Alcohol withdrawal symptoms?"

"Yes. Almost all of my problems can be directly related to alcohol withdrawal. With extreme agitation and absent a sedative, I have to keep drinking."

Oscar leaned forward and lectured, "You just referred to an episode of delirium tremens or what's commonly referred to as DTs. That alone is diagnostic of alcoholism. Social drinkers don't have DTs."

I rolled my eyes while responding, "Granted. However, it happened only once and it was before I was prescribed a sedative called Ativan. I would prefer Valium or Librium, but it is impossible to find any doctor to prescribe either, and I will not buy pills on the street. I am not a drug addict! However, Ativan is effective in treating alcohol withdrawal. With no appreciable withdrawal, there is no need for morning drinking that sometimes results in a binge."

"I see. You detox yourself with drugs."

"A drug. Not drugs. To be precise, it is medication prescribed by a psychiatrist at a VA hospital to treat post-traumatic stress disorder with recurrent panic attacks caused by my experiences in the Persian Gulf War."

Oscar inquired, "Were you in combat?"

"No, but I saw a lot of shit."

Oscar picked up a long red pen and scribbled something on his notepad while stating, "We will return to your military service at some point. But regarding the anti-anxiety medication that you are taking, prescribed medication does sound better than drug, I would have to agree. You do know that there is a significant mortality rate for untreated DTs?"

"Yes. Untreated DTs."

"But that's why you are here. Whoever made this appointment said you just had an episode of severe alcohol withdrawal."

"That would be my wife. She exaggerates. But yes, I did have a bit of difficulty coming off the last one, but it was the first time in years that I was without my sedative. I didn't even have any booze to taper off with. That is exceedingly rare. Normally, I have a pint of vodka in my coat or trunk of my car and a supply of Ativan on hand."

"You could have chosen not to drink knowing you did not have your detox drug."

"It is interesting that you call Ativan a "detox drug" rather than a prescribed anti-anxiety agent."

"Agent. That does have a nice ring to it. And is the agent prescribed by a doctor for the purpose of self-detoxification from alcohol withdrawal on a recurrent basis?"

"Of course not. Let's get something straight Oscar. While the asterisk is valid under even superficial scrutiny, I did concede that I'm an alcoholic. But the important point here is that I am a functional alcoholic. As long as I have my sedative, I'm fine—it nips any potential binge right in the bud. Moreover, I can keep my periodic drinking under sufficient control to minimize any unpleasant residuals. Not just intermittent manageability; I'm talking about the ongoing manageable life of a functional alcoholic."

With a wry smile Oscar replied, "There's an oxymoron if I ever heard one: ongoing, manageable alcoholism. We'll try and unpack that a little later, but first, can you please relax and explain what you mean by blackouts?"

"Sure. My friend Lou just brought up an incident yesterday. With my wife out of town, we were sitting in my kitchen drinking before we hit the bars to save money, but after drinking more than I planned to, I momentarily dozed off. When I opened my eyes, I asked, 'Lou, did we go out and come back?'

Lou answered, 'No, we haven't gone out yet.'

I said, "Thank God."

"And you don't remember that Freddie?"

"Not a thing."

"Lou also brought up an episode in a bar. I was trying to talk to two women sitting alone at a table and I fell out of my chair. He was driving and ready to leave; it was about 3 am. Lou walked over and looking down, asked me if I was ready to leave. I lifted my head and answered 'No. I wana hang around for a couple of more drinks.'"

Oscar said through a smirk, "I see. In other words, in addition to bouts of gross intoxication, blackouts of hours' duration, and severe alcohol withdrawal symptoms, you have identified a 4th characteristic of alcoholism: craving."

"Let's examine the entire record Oscar. I never lost a job because of drinking. I did have a close call after being found drunk on the floor in my office with an empty bottle of vodka on my desk, but I went straight to detox and they were very understanding about it. That binge was the result of my wife locking me out of our house and my not having a sedative. I felt humiliated returning to work with my tail between my legs. That kind of thing gets around the agency in a hurry."

"I can see how that would make for lively water cooler conversation."

"You can say that again. Still, I must say with all honesty that my boss would say I am a cracker-jack lawyer, and my ex-wife and soon to be ex-wife number 2 would say I was not a bad husband overall. And a darn good parent."

"Soon to be ex number 2?"

"Yeah. She has been threatening a divorce for the past year, and we have only been married for two years. But it's not just my drinking. To tell you the truth, she can be a real pain in the ass and it would be nice not to hear the nagging about having a couple of drinks."

"Ahh yes, the proverbial couple of drinks. It's never one or three or four or 10; it is always a couple. Why are you here Freddie?"

"I agreed to do this because of my wife. But I'm coming here in good faith and with an open mind."

Oscar wrote a few more notes while asking, "Is it safe to say that when you drink you can't always predict the outcome?"

"Do you mind if I stand?"

"Not at all."

I stood and began pacing back and forth while raising my voice, "Can't always predict the outcome. Who the hell can say always? You can walk out of here and get hit by a bus.

"While it's true that I have been mugged many times, most of that happened years ago when I was young and very careless. On one occasion it was all very innocent. I was living in Sheepshead Bay, Brooklyn and after a night out on the town, I took the "D" train from the city all the way through Brooklyn, but I fell asleep and missed my stop."

"Were you drunk?"

"Plastered. A cop woke me up at the last stop, Coney Island, so I went around to the other side. I only had 3 stops to go, but I fell asleep again and woke up in the Bronx."

"Awakened by another cop?"

"No. I awoke to morning sunlight streaming through the subway car window. On my way back, I started getting the shakes so I got off the train, even though I knew I was in a rough part of the South Bronx."

"What part isn't?"

"In acute withdrawal, I have no choice. In any event, all my fears melted away after a few drinks in this very dark bar with some great 60's Do-Wop music on the jukebox. But when I left two guys followed me out. One of the thugs hit me in the right knee with a lead pipe while the other punk was taking off my new suede jacket. My knee blew up to twice its size; I had a limp for at least two months."

Oscar observed, "He could have hit you in the head."

"It's really unfortunate that I started having this withdrawal problem so young. That has led to almost all of my alcohol-related problems. I think the withdrawal syndrome, like alcoholism itself, is at least in part genetic. But there is a solution."

"To alcoholism?"

"I was referring to alcohol withdrawal. The solution is a sedative."

Oscar leaned forward over his desk while saying, "That's like giving someone aspirin to treat a fever when the real problem is pneumonia. If you don't treat the underlying pneumonia, the fever will come back and you will end up with more serious systemic complications. You need to treat the underlying alcoholism Freddie. You won't have withdrawal if you don't drink."

"Bravo Oscar. I suppose it takes years of training and obtaining your certification in counseling to grasp that pearl of wisdom."

"I'm not the one in the hot seat Freddie. Do you have any history of alcohol-related legal problems?"

"A few arrests for being drunk and disorderly, but they happened when I was young and slightly out of control. I also had a couple of DWIs, but one of those was because of a busted tail light a block from home.

"Oscar asked with another sneer, "A busted tail light?"

"Correct."

Oscar, grim faced, leaned further forward and said, "You got the DWI because you were drunk. They don't arrest people for a broken tail light."

"True. But I would not have had the DWI but for the busted tail light. They pulled me over and the first thing the cop said was that my tail light was not working. I don't even think he suspected I was drunk until I breathed on him."

"It's hard to avoid breathing."

"Well Oscar, you do get a lot more careful with advancing age. At least I do. I believe with some extra vigilance, I could be classified as a borderline alcoholic. That is, by incorporating a series of safeguards that I will get to momentarily."

"Safeguards. I look forward to hearing your strategies for an alcoholic to safely drink and stop the progression of the disease."

"Everything is relative Oscar. There are few guarantees in life. I'm talking percentages or odds in my favor."

"With respect to driving drunk, such episodes have been few and far between, but I must eliminate that risk entirely. I want to look into the possibility of whether you can get a Breath Alcohol Ignition Interlock Device installed in your car without having any court order to do so."

"I don't think so Freddie."

"I'll bet that can be arranged. Money talks. I'm looking for a semblance of control—a way to minimize the collateral damage. I can't stand all of the absolutes people apply to alcoholics, especially these holier than thou AAs. It's a hell-of-a lot more nuanced."

Oscar responded, "We will eventually talk about AA."

"Fuck AA."

I was still pacing back and forth and quite animated. Oscar sat back in his chair with his hands clasped behind his head. He seemed awfully relaxed; I wondered whether he was on drugs.

"O.K. Freddie. Can you give me some examples of these nuances as you put it?"

I sat back down and took a couple of deep breaths. "Certainly. Maybe now we can get somewhere. I can drink with a significantly reduced risk of unpleasantness by following a few simple steps:

A. Leave my car keys at home, hidden in the attic or better yet have a Breath Alcohol Ignition Device installed in my car. I need to look into that."

Oscar interrupted, "Get the one where you have to breathe into it every 5 minutes or your car stops."

"B. Do not drink with my wife at home. Her work takes her out of town a lot, and at other times I can always say I'm going on a golfing trip or attending a legal conference. I have many opportunities to pick my spots. There's really no need to drink and try to hide it coming in the door. I have not been very successful doing that. She can see it in my face or sniff it out a mile away."

Oscar rudely interposed, "It is interesting that you used the word semblance of control, which is defined as an appearance of control. In other words, it looks like control, but it's not."

"I wasn't an English major Oscar. I think you know what I mean. Sufficient control to minimize risks."

"It sounds like you have to lie to your wife, to include saying you are traveling for things like a work-related conference or golf when you are not going to do that at all. You're planning a weekend drunk."

"I'm not trying to be a saint. All you AA's say we are not saints, don't you? Now, may I continue with my analysis?"

"By all means Fred."

"Freddie."

"OK."

I continued,

"C. Do not drink alone. Rather, imbibe with a friend who likes to drink a lot but does not get trashed;

"D. Hire a big guy—a body guard if you will—who will be out front of whatever bar I'm drinking in but looking through the big window, keeping me within seeing distance. And in doing so, he can walk in and pluck me out of whatever jam I might get myself into. Better yet, let's make it a driver-bodyguard, which would eliminate the need for A.

"Finally, and most importantly,

E. Always have a pint of top-shelf vodka and a sufficient amount of a sedative at the ready for detox purposes.

"If I had the money, I would also have a nurse. In fact, as ridiculous as that may sound, that would be money well spent to help prevent the possibility of an accidental overdose of booze and pills. While an OD is extremely unlikely, I'll admit that I sometimes keep drinking after I take a sedative in the morning."

"You would have a tough time explaining the nurse to your wife. And it would have to be a traveling nurse."

"Well Oscar, having a big man on my side would virtually eliminate any problems out on the town, to include potential muggings, leaving an expensive coat in the bar, and fights. Unlike your daily lush, I can pick and choose my spots."

"All of this sounds like a lot of work?"

"Not really."

"Any prior contact with AA Freddie?"

"Yes. There's no question that AA is the best way to go to get sober if that is what you want, but they can be a bit cultish. And let's face it, there are also a lot of assholes in AA. Don't get me wrong. I'm sure a lot of people are helped if they stay with it, but it's definitely not for me; not at this point in my life."

"How long did you go to meetings?"

"About a week."

"That long."

"Long enough. I can't stand some of these old timers; big blowhards preening around the rooms, beating their breasts. They love to hear themselves talk and think they are anointed gurus with all the answers. AA is their whole life. I find it very sad."

"Don't you think you need to take a longer look? Maybe shop around for a meeting you are comfortable with?"

"Look Oscar, I have reached a different level of consciousness in my life. I'm more mature based upon many life experiences. It's my view that after all I have been through, I can drink relatively safely, provided certain precautions are solidly in place. While it is true that there is a part of me that still wants to drink with abandon, the older, wiser, more sensible part stresses caution."

"Tell me more about those safeguards."

"Sure. I would like to expand on my idea of hiring a big guy to follow me around while I drink. It is not an absurd idea for someone with my history. In these tough economic times, it wouldn't be hard to find someone who would work for 10 bucks an hour. That seems to be the going rate for a lot of things in Buffalo, including difficult work like painting houses, or even certain types of construction as long as it's under the table."

"Would you pay your big man under the table?"

"Come on Oscar. Next you will be asking me about FICA taxes."

"That was my next question."

"You're a riot. To continue, having the big man with me from 9 pm to 4 am is not going to cost all that much when you consider what I would end up avoiding, namely those costly mishaps. In the long run, I would save

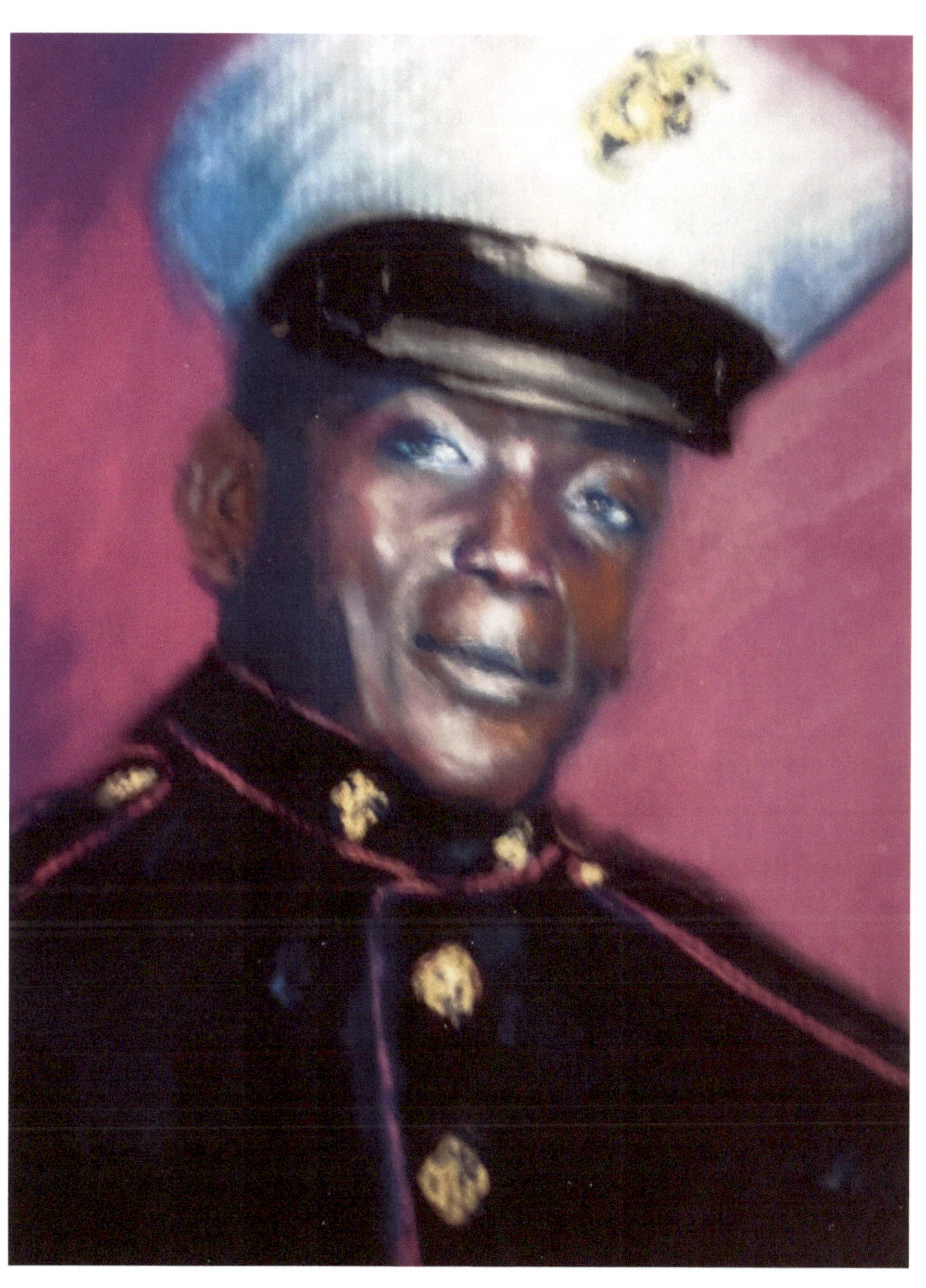

Charles
Vietnam
NYC VA Regional Office Museum

money. I am absolutely certain of it."

"Mishaps?"

"Muggings with loss of wallets, watches, suit coats, and overcoats for example. Also fights and leaving money on bars or having it drop out of my pocket. Of course, this would assume that my man would pick it up and give it to me. For ten bucks an hour, I suppose it is just as likely that he would take the dough. Still, I think there is great potential if I think this through, to include finding someone trustworthy, perhaps recommended by a reliable source. I would insist on a thorough interview. There would have to be a certain comfort level."

"Of course. Every alcoholic with a car should have a big man/driver."

"In a perfect world—absolutely. But even for those that can just barely afford it, you can't put a price tag on that kind of insurance. Just the thought of me ending up in prison, living day to day with the knowledge that I killed someone driving drunk sends chills up my spine. In my view, having a driver is a great idea."

Oscar replied, "And he must be a sober big man who's light on his feet."

I ignored the sarcasm. On a roll, my voice rose and leaning forward, my hands went into action as I continued, "Shifting now to the bodyguard part of the equation, the driver could park in front of or near where I am doing my drinking. I probably average about 5 or 6 bars during a night on the town. He could stay in front of the place on foot and glance in frequently. As I said earlier, if he spots a problem, he can intervene on my behalf. Thereafter, he can bring me to a safer bar. In certain joints, my bodyguard could be sitting at a table sipping a coke. He would have a clear view to where I am sitting at the bar. A big man: ready, willing, and able."

"Would you bring the big man on your weekend get-a-ways?"

"No. I would have to draw the line there. A plane ticket and a separate hotel room—I certainly wouldn't want him in my room—would be a bit much. However, my plan for these weekends will always include a drinking friend who is not as bad as me."

"Not as bad as you? That's a pretty low bar."

"Out of town benders are generally safer anyway. There is no car or wife in the equation, and I can stick with high end cocktail lounges. Why spend a lot of money flying to a city just to end up in a shithole where I might get my ass kicked.

"But on home turf, I could also ask my big man to periodically come up behind me and whisper certain things like, 'Slow down boss'; or 'Take your time boss as you are already pretty drunk'; or "Watch out for that guy with a beard at the other end of the bar.' Or even, 'That pretty lady at the end of the bar is giving you the eye.' I think I miss that kind of thing sometimes, and it looks like I will be single again soon. There are so many invaluable things a big man on your side can do for you. And it's not exactly manual labor."

Oscar shot back, "Following you around for a night sounds pretty taxing to me."

Oscar's snide remarks were becoming intolerable. I raised my voice stating, "If I'm a big guy looking to make some extra money, this would be a great job. I go to nice places and he can soak up that atmosphere, an ambiance that he might not otherwise be privileged to experience. In a small way, I'd be contributing to society."

Oscar interjected, "Community service!"

"Home in Buffalo, there will be some dives of course. That's where I would need him the most. And after last call? I go down quietly. I would only want to have my man see that I got into the house safely, so an extra half hour or so might be a good idea."

Oscar counseled, "You would have to have a shift change with the second wide-awake guy there to watch you every time you got up to relieve yourself. Accidents in the home are quite common. For example, head trauma from a fall is one of many reasons why the alcoholic has a significantly lower life expectancy."

"Good point Oscar. That's what happened to Williams Holden, who by the way was a very successful actor and therefore a functional alcoholic. I'm glad I'm talking about this as it flushes out good ideas. My big guy would probably have to watch me eat now that I think of it. I usually do that after coming home drunk. I could wear an adult diaper. All of this may sound pretty nuts to some people, but it makes perfect sense to anyone who drinks like me. And when factoring everything in, it would end up saving a lot of money and misery."

"It does sound cost effective at that," Oscar replied. "Of course, you could save even more money by not drinking."

"Not on the table. I am simply not convinced that I am nothing more than a functional alcoholic who gets drunk a couple of times a month and that's nowhere near the kind of daily drinking a lot of alcoholics do. They can't even go a day without the sauce. You must have met many of those types. I can go weeks without a drop, months if absolutely necessary."

"Months Freddie? If you are by yourself?"

"Well weeks. A couple of weeks if I have to."

Oscar turned somber. "Many alcoholics can space out their binges. However, alcoholism is a progressive disease. They inevitably drink more often and are obsessed about it between sprees. We call them dry drunks.

And they are still at a very high risk of serious if not fatal complications. It makes it rather difficult to have a serene life."

"Who the hell lives a serene life Oscar? AA's? They are full of shit. I'm only entering my 40s. The way I figure it, I can go another 10 or 15 years before throwing in the towel. In addition to not being close to a daily drinker, I can accomplish most if not all of the numerous things that I need to do, like work and have quality time with family."

"An active alcoholic having quality time with his family you say? That is oxymoron number two."

I paid no attention to Oscar's lame attempts at mockery. "I hear a lot of alcoholics talk about drinking straight from the bottle. I very rarely do that. I heard a guy in an AA meeting say he sat in front of his TV drinking a cheap bottle of whiskey. Thereafter, he would pass out and wake up looking at the test pattern. How pathetic! I drink mixed drinks in bars with music playing and meet interesting people. I don't like being categorized. So many people want to pigeonhole you. People, including alcoholics are far more complicated Oscar."

Turning serious again, Oscar warned, "It sounds like despite your normally having a sedative to detox yourself, you have been caught a number of times without it, sometimes resulting in near fatal withdrawal or uncontrollable, potentially lethal binges; or even with Ativan, often drinking on top of it, raising the risk of overdose. You're fucked any way you turn."

"Near fatal, lethal, overdosing; such hyperbole Oscar. There have been very few uncontrollable binges. I think approaching this in a systematic way, I can make sure everything is in place to prevent such complications of withdrawal, to include uncontrollable binges. I can keep Ativan in two places: a vial in my pocket and a stash at home."

"I thought you said you weren't buying drugs on the street?"

"I'm not. I think I can get a higher dose from the VA, although I would need a different psychiatrist. The one I have now has even hinted at weaning me off, which scares the hell out of me. But I buy it from a friend who only takes it PRN."

"Whenever necessary."

"That's right. And he does just that, so he always has a good supply on hand. He can also use the extra money. It's a win-win."

"But Freddie, if you only take it for detox purposes, why don't you have an extra supply?"

"I never said I only take it for detoxification from alcohol purposes. I take it as prescribed for anxiety and sometimes I need extra."

"Why extra?"

I stood up, pointed toward the window, and hollered, "Because I have to live with someone who can be a real bitch. I also need more when I'm coming off a drunk. So, let me admit here and now, I buy some extra Ativan from my buddy, but it's not in the street. He's not a drug dealer. I'm his only client."

"You do know that you are in danger of overdosing when you are on a high dose of a sedative on a daily basis, take more when coming off a drunk, and sometimes drink on top of that?"

"I'm also on the maximum dose of an anti-depressant called Doxepin, 300 mg. at night. My shrink says no one can go any higher than that."

"Lord have mercy Freddie! You're out of your mind drinking on top of all of that."

"But here again Oscar, you have to look at the individual and not paint everything with a broad brush. I have been taking these medications for many years and have built up a tolerance."

"But you take more Ativan as you are detoxing?"

"Yes, but spaced out. If I drink on a work night, which is rare, I can still go to work with mild sedation. I hate to go to my office like that as I have an increased startle response, but I function all right. I'm even steady enough sometimes to go out and get a sandwich for lunch. Without a sedative, I end up drinking from a pint in a bathroom stall; for a guy who loves bars, it is a bit depressing drinking while sitting on a toilet. But I get in and out quickly after a couple of gulps, although I got caught once."

Oscar inquired, "Caught?"

"Yes. This asshole Murphy opened up my stall by mistake. I didn't lock it. It was embarrassing as I was taking a full slug out of a pint of vodka."

Oscar replied, "While sitting on a toilet; I suppose that got around the agency too."

"I didn't sweat it much. Murph's a boozer and everybody knows it. He has that flushed swollen face with shiny stretched skin and a red nose like W. C. Fields. If he opened his mouth— Oh Baby. Talk about the pot calling the kettle black!"

"But Freddie, regarding your mixing of pills and alcohol, you must know that one drug potentiates the other. For example, if you combine 1 mg. of Ativan and one shot of booze, it is like taking two shots of booze. Maybe three shots."

"Two shots at most. I have done the research and looked at this thing from every angle Oscar. I have not come close to overdosing, and I don't do drugs. We are not taking about heroin or cocaine. In my experience, not yours or anyone else's but mine, I have never come close to overdosing on anything."

"You have no idea what your blood levels of booze and pills are when you pass out—you might be very close to acute respiratory failure. There is an area in the brain that controls respiration; if it is overwhelmed by alcohol, it's lights out for good. And you're leaving out blackouts, a common occurrence, when your forehead slams against the top of the bar."

I shot back, "When that happens, I'm quite sure they wake me up and shut me off. Passing out is not overdosing and if I do pass out, I must awaken easy enough; I don't recall any ambulances or hospitalizations. I never got such a bill in the mail."

"Yes. You don't recall. That's the point. But let's leave the question of mixing a sedative with alcohol, which does result in accidental overdoses all the—"

"Please Oscar, let's dispense with lecture on ODs; that is irrelevant."

"All right. Let's return to your various ideas to, as you put it, keep some semblance of control of your drinking. How is that working for you?"

"On the average, it's somewhere between usual and total control. Simply put, a functional alcoholic is able, with help, to minimize the risk of harm. I will admit that I haven't actually incorporated many of these ideas yet."

"Like what?"

"For example, my buddy Phil has recommended I ask every bartender for a tall glass of water and to drink it between every couple of drinks. I think this is a brilliant idea. There's no question I often drink too fast and all that booze overwhelms the brain sensors. I end up in a blackout way too early in the game. The water would slow everything down. The whole idea for a lot of alcoholics is to get as fucked up as quickly as possible. For me, it is not just about the booze. I enjoy the ride, to include expensive cocktail lounges without the riffraff to classic blue-collar bars with character—one might say I'm bicultural in that regard—and meeting fascinating people in both venues."

"Fascinating people you say. I'll bet. Have you tried the water idea?"

"To be honest, I have either forgotten to do it, or in a couple of cases after having a few, I just thought fuck the water. That's one of the things my big man can do for me. He could say, 'Drink that water even if you don't want to,' and I wouldn't mind if he says so forcefully.

"I also try and have a game plan Oscar. I write an outline with notes before setting forth. For example, I'm meeting my friend Phil in Manhattan for a 3-day weekend beginning this Friday. He loves the bar room atmosphere as much as I do. I don't think he's an alcoholic. He drinks a lot but he stays on his feet."

"Stays on his feet. An even lower bar—no pun intended."

I tried to disregard Oscar's ridicule, but I have to admit it got on my nerves. Nevertheless, I soldiered on. "I have made a list of places to go with a timeline for the entire three-day weekend. My plan will ensure some memorable experiences and most importantly, it significantly lowers the risk of disagreeable events."

Oscar leaned forward with his bushy black eyebrows raised—Grouchoesque—and softly said, "I'm all ears."

"Here it is in a nutshell. We will be arriving from different cities to meet at a Times Square hotel, cheap but centrally located, at noon on Thursday, August 16. I'll take care of the early check-in fee if necessary. There's a Yankee game that afternoon, which would be a perfect way to begin. With a starting time of 1:05 pm, we would get there no later than the second inning. I figure on no more than 5 or 6 beers at the game. That would not get me drunk at all; simply feeling good. After the game, we could stop at a bar near the stadium that has character and is relatively safe. You don't want to get off the beaten path in the South Bronx."

"Especially that bar where you got whacked by a metal bar in the knee and lost your new suede jacket."

"I am mindful of the Santayana quote: 'Those who cannot remember the past are condemned to repeat it.' "

"With your blackout history, you can't remember—"

"Please Oscar. As I was saying, a couple of drinks before heading downtown—no more than that—is a must to keep the jag afloat. Next, we take the subway all of the way downtown to the Wall Street area, so by the time we get there my blood alcohol level would be low, but not to a degree to eliminate the buzz. This is extremely important."

Oscar kept shifting in his chair, like he couldn't get comfortable, and he repeatedly looked down at his notes.

In a louder voice, I continued, "Phil has a busy dental practice, but he finds time to be a day trader. I don't give a fuck about the stock market, but it would be an experience for me too, mixing with all of these white-collar criminals that are robbing people blind with their insider trading."

"Sounds good on paper."

"I'm not done. After a couple of mixed drinks and some interesting conversation, I will walk Phil through lower Manhattan into Chinatown. We can have another drink or two in a restaurant with one of those small glitzy bars with a beautiful Asian barmaid. I worked nearby many years ago and did a lot of drinking in Chinatown. I'll bet there are people still around that will remember me."

Oscar posited, "I'll bet there are."

"Then we would cross Canal Street into Little Italy and have dinner with wine at an outdoor café. This is a sure winner, sitting at a table on Mulberry Street while people watching. I will have sausage and peppers with a little pasta with tomato sauce on the side and wine. I'll bet we reminisce about prior joint escapades. Phil is very good at filling in the blanks, although he does have brownouts sometimes. He can get a little loud with half a load on too and those outdoor tables are very close together. At any rate, by the time we would head back uptown, I would be high but not drunk. There is no worry about Phil as he has a tolerance that I envy."

"I'm impressed. You even have what you are going to talk about in the plan."

"Phil can help me out with the wine selection. My drink of choice is vodka. But pasta in Little Italy demands a fine wine."

"Of course."

Oscar, leaning back in his chair while pushing his glasses with his right index finger on to the top of his bald head further remarked, "And such detail, right down to the sausage and peppers."

"That's right. And here's the real beauty of the plan. The breaking up of the afternoon and early evening with the train ride and our intermittent walking are important as the blood alcohol level continues to drop. That will prevent gross intoxication way too early in the evening, but not allowing too much time to elapse as I would lose that pleasingly plastered feeling. It's all about keeping that jag afloat. We will cab it uptown without fucking around with the subway."

"You don't want that blood alcohol level to drop too much."

"Exactly. We could cap off the evening at the Café Carlyle. Will I be drunk at the end of the night? There's no question about it. Frankly, that's the goal. But by spacing out my drinks, I will remember and enjoy the entire experience. And I'm bringing my white dinner jacket."

"A nice touch."

"I think so. I love dressing well and going to places with class in Manhattan, where it is safe. You tell me Oscar and try to be honest. Take your AA and alcohol counselor hats off, be objective, and tell me whether this plan would minimize any complications?"

Oscar frowned and said while shaking his head, "It sounds like you are romanticizing your next drunk, but such thoughts are delusional as they have no factual basis. In other words, you may be picturing yourself in a fancy place with your white dinner jacket perfectly articulating, 'Another cocktail my dear?' when in reality you'll be soused and slurring your speech. Most women don't like talking to someone who is grossly intoxicated."

"Poppycock."

I heard a buzz from Oscar's watch indicating the session was over. As we rose together and shook hands, Oscar sternly advised, "Sobriety is about changing your thinking Fred, but I can see you have no desire to stay sober. With all of your delusional thinking, I don't see you living very long. You will end up alone with end stage alcoholism with its myriad of physical and mental complications. And that is a miserable way to exist."

"End stage Oscar? Balderdash! I'll soon be wining and dining in Manhattan with my pal Phil."

On my way out the door, a thought came into my brain that was perhaps more significant than anything I had ever considered in the context of functional alcoholism; it was startling and profound yet simple and right in front of my nose. I have no idea why I never thought of it.

Stepping back into the office and looking at the back of Oscar's bald head rising from his notes, I said while standing proudly like a soldier ready for battle, "One other thing Oscar and this is critical. Even assuming that I have some regrets in the morning after every night of drinking—and I'm not conceding that this is the case for a moment as the first couple of hours alone are enjoyable—but for the sake of argument, accepting everything you are saying is true, during the period of time in-between drunks, and this is at a minimum one week averaging closer to two, I thoroughly enjoy planning and fantasizing about my next spree. How it turns out is almost irrelevant. Take my pending long weekend I just talked about; if it doesn't work out as planned, that doesn't take away for a second the time I was fantasizing about it. And that my friend is serenity; it is what you AAs call the pure joy of living. Daydreaming about sprees; in my case, that's a lot of time, much more than the actual drinking. Indeed, it's most of my adult life. Serenity? You bet I've got it and more often than your average ex-boozer sitting in a church basement drinking shitty coffee out of Styrofoam cups and talking to a bunch of boring stiffs."

I concluded my soliloquy with great passion by raising my right hand with extended index finger in the air and proclaiming, "And you, my wife; not even God Almighty can take that away from me. Abstinence and A.A meetings you say? I would rather be sacrificed on the altar of Bacchus!"

Still standing behind Oscar and looking at the back of his shiny dome, I watched him shaking his head back and forth. I made a crisp about-face and marched with confidence with a broad smile down the long hall, knowing that I had won Round One from a formidable opponent.

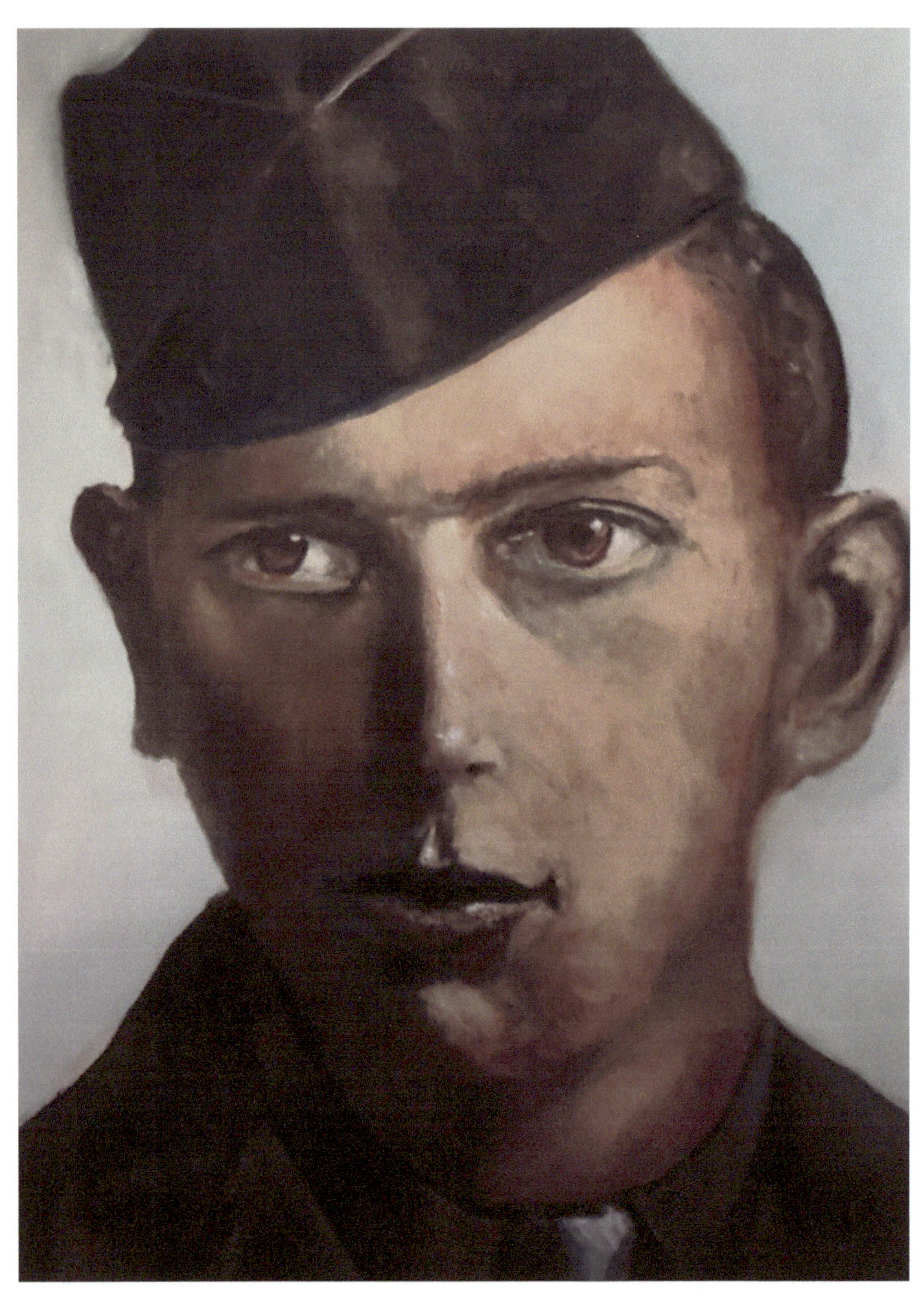

Roy
KIA, WW II
NYC VA Regional Office Museum

***

Freddie and Oscar: Round II

After arriving for my second appointment with Oscar, he was on his desk phone and motioned for me to sit down. His skin tight, bright red polo shirt purposely increased the level of intimidation or so he thought. I was on to him after that first session.

When he hung up the phone, he sternly asked, "Before we get started Fred, I must ask you, "Have you ever thought of suicide?"

"It's crossed my mind. I think that's probably true of everyone."

Oscar answered, "Actually it's not. Have you thought about it recently? Do you ever have a plan to kill yourself? In other words, do you think of, for example, intentionally overdosing with pills and booze?"

"No. If I was seriously considering suicide, I would go on a long bender in Europe first, starting in Spain and working my way across the continent. Eating tapas with cold beer into the wee hours in Madrid; sipping wine in an outdoor café in Paris; relaxing on the Grand Canal in Venice with a Martini; sunning on one of the Greek Islands while drinking shots of Ouzo with calamari so fresh they are jumping on your plate—I don't understand why anyone wouldn't take a trip like that before offing themselves. Max out your credit cards if need be. Besides, there's still a lot of life I want to live, more things to do. And I have a daughter to think about."

"Your history of drinking indicates that you are committing a not so slow suicide, but I wanted to get the question of pending suicidal ideation clarified."

"Of course, Oscar. It's probably on some list or protocol that you need to follow. I get it. Check the no box."

Oscar half grinned and said, "Go ahead with your New York City story. I'm dying to hear it."

I sat on the edge of the wooden chair directly across from Oscar leaning back in his dark green, fake leather chair and began sharing my New York City weekend. Surprisingly, he let me tell it without any interruptions.

"I arrived in mid-town Manhattan and bought two pints of rum, along with a ten pack of cheap airline bottles of vodka, in a Times Square liquor store. No need to go top shelf in treating my morning alcohol withdrawal symptoms, I reasoned. Some disheveled guy followed me while asking, "Can you buy me a pint?" Not a quarter or a buck like in the old days. A pint with demand in his voice. The nerve! I sadly reflected it was just one more sign of the coarsening of the culture. I did waiver as he appeared to have the jitters, thinking about giving the bum one of my small bottles of vodka, but I didn't want to enable him.

"After slipping a hotel clerk a 20-dollar bill for an early check-in, I was in my room and unpacked by 12:30 pm, anxiously looking at my watch every couple of minutes. I was sipping a rum and coke while looking down at the traffic on Eighth Avenue ten floors below. Every other car was a yellow cab and each time one stopped in front of the hotel and someone got out, I looked to see if it was Phil. I didn't want to get started before he arrived—that was not part of my best laid plan—but I made another drink while thinking I might as well relax.

"As I was pacing back and forth, there was a welcome knock on the door. Phil arrived at 1:30 pm, just after I consumed my 4th mixed drink to unwind. While feeling relaxed, I began having ambivalent feelings about taking a subway to Yankee stadium.

It was a moot point because the first thing Phil said upon arrival was. "I don't feel like rushing around trying to get to the game." He kept looking at my pint of rum.

"Phil had two rum and cokes which took care of my pint and smoked a joint. I opened an airline bottle of vodka and had a 5th drink, along with a few hits of his weed and we were on our way. I noticed that Phil had been working out; we are both tall and thin, but Phil is muscular with a full head of red hair that he left mussed up as is the style. While immersed in the usual flow of people walking on 7th Ave., I remember being mildly concerned about my stash of morning booze already getting low before the first morning after. Nevertheless, I was comforted in the knowledge that there were liquor stores all over Times Square and early opening bars to drink if I was so inclined. I even thought a bar might be a better way to go. Early morning drinking in a dark bar was a pleasing thought; no pretense—anyone present at that hour in a dive would be an alcoholic and I always found that liberating. And believe it or not Oscar, I have met some interesting characters in such a setting."

Oscar was stretched back in his chair as far as he could go without flipping over and his eyes were half closed. I stopped talking and there was silence for a few seconds, but he suddenly sat up and said, "Interesting? Let's hear it. Give it to me straight Freddie."

"Thank-you Oscar. I thought you might be asleep. To continue, the rest of the evening was a blackout for me. In fact, the whole weekend was no more than a blur. We never made it to Wall Street, Chinatown, or that outdoor café in Little Italy for sausage and peppers with wine. One of the few memories I had was waking up on a bench along Central Park South at 2 am. I lost a lot of money; it must have been around $300, because

I was using a credit card to keep the cash in reserve. It was possible it simply fell out of my pocket as the bills were probably rolled up in a ball. When drinking, I have a bad habit of pulling everything out of my wallet to pay for something and then stuffing what's left in my pocket. It is also conceivable that some scum bag robbed me. I need to give more thought to bringing a big man with me on the road.

"The only other problem was that my white dinner jacket had wine and grass stains. The splotch of wine on my lapel was not shocking, but the large grass stain on the back certainly was. I must have ended up stretched out on some grassy knoll in Central Park before I found the bench or I may have been dragged in the park and mugged. But I quickly dismissed such unpleasant thoughts since I couldn't do anything about it, and there were two more days and evenings to go. Accordingly, I suited up with confidence the next morning after a generous dose of a tranquilizer washed down with a coffee-vodka mix."

After concluding my weekend in Manhattan summary, Oscar sat in silence, staring at me for a full minute. It was rather unnerving frankly. He finally stood up. While pacing the room with an overly dramatic use of his hands, he cried, "I think that is the best example of craving I have ever heard, and I have been around an awful lot of alcoholics over three decades. What I mean is you had a strategy—an incredibly detailed plan. And as soon as you started drinking, all bets were off. You went on a binge, drinking until you were plastered, in a blackout, and then kept drinking beyond that without doing one thing on that list of yours."

I calmly responded, "Yes and no Oscar. Regarding my plan, I would have to concede that what seemed foreseeable became unpredictable after having too many too soon. AA says the first drink gets you drunk? Bullshit. The first 5 drinks consumed rapidly gets you well on your way too soon, but there was no binge so settle down. I drank the three days I planned to with my buddy and that was it."

Oscar sat down, leaned over his desk and barked, "With your buddy? You just got through saying you ended up alone. And it was a 4-day binge."

"Four?"

"You must have drunk that 4th morning, didn't you? In other words, after the third night or more precisely third day and night of drinking, you drank the next morning to calm your shakes."

I knew I had him. "Correct. I always have to do that or take double doses of my sedative, and I have been very candid about it. It's either that or severe alcohol withdrawal. But that was not a full day of drinking. I did not even get drunk. I'm glad you brought it up. I drank to steady my nerves but did not get drunk on the 4th day as I had to catch my flight. That's 25% of the long weekend. Kind of blows your theory that alcoholism is always manifested by craving."

Oscar, looking exasperated, threw his hands up and said, "You're a hard nut to crack Fred."

"Freddie."

"What you are describing is not social drinking. Can't you see that?"

I retorted, "Yes, it is. It is the most sociable thing I can do. I am three times more genial. And I absolutely love lounges where you can dress up, especially in a tux or a white dinner jacket. Maybe even an ascot without people judging you as being pretentious."

"You mean the white dinner jacket with the wine and grass stains?"

"The fresh from the cleaner's white dinner jacket Oscar."

"And the ascot? Is that the thing you wear around your neck in place of a tie? I'm thinking David Niven."

"The dashing David Niven," I responded. "I could wear an ascot to lots of places in Manhattan and not feel like an asshole; lounges where you can be who you want to be. It's about sophistication. And pretension gets an unfair rap. I like a little pretension in others."

I continued with the dramatic yet thoughtful oration with use of my right hand for emphasis. "I often find pretension amusing in men and endearing with women of means. They are also locked into their world by genes, environmental factors, and culture with no way out. I sometimes have sympathy for the upper crust. When all is said and done, aren't we all just trying to get through another day the best way we know how?"

I might have been mistaken, but I thought I saw a tear welled up in Oscar's right eye.

I concluded, "In most places, and this certainly includes Buffalo, if you dress nice people think you are a snob or simply an asshole. It is a sad commentary on our contemporary culture if you ask me."

"Why can't you wear your white dinner jacket and ascot without drinking?"

"It's not the same Oscar. There has to be wine or a martini to fill out the picture."

"To fill out your fantasy. What good does it do to be in a tux or wearing an ascot when you are in a blackout and get rolled?"

"I can find ways to prevent such a level of inebriation. That's what this counseling is all about for me. Besides, there is always a window of tranquility before the blackout."

"You're delusional Freddie."

"I don't think so. But if you want to know what fuels my desire, the sophisticated lounge is a big part of it.”

Oscar looked down and opened up a blue book on his desk. After putting his black framed reading glasses on, he said in a monotonous tone, raising his eyes above his glasses to look at me at the end of every sentence, “On page 30 in the Big Book, the bible of Alcoholics Anonymous, there is a passage I would like to read to you. The idea that somehow, someday he will control and enjoy his drinking is the great obsession of every abnormal drinker. The persistence of this illusion is astonishing. Many pursue it into the gates of insanity or death.”

I shook my head and exclaimed, “Gates of insanity? I have known a lot of alcoholics and not one went insane. Not one. Someone should revise that AA book of yours. I have no doubt that, everything else being equal, one’s life expectancy is reduced, but I’ll bet most alcoholics die from diseases that have nothing to do with their alcoholism. How about both of us telling the truth and stop with the theatrics.”

Oscar calmly replied, “Some alcoholics do die of old age, but they have miserable lives.”

“How the hell do you know they have miserable lives Oscar? Does someone from AA follow them around? This is exactly what I’m talking about. Frankly, I’m a hell of a lot more miserable sober.

“And regarding your quote, I have never had an obsession to be a normal drinker. I want to get drunk. If I have a delusion, and I’m not conceding I do, it would be that I am a functional alcoholic. That is, getting drunk once a week without any appreciable collateral damage. I can’t think of one important thing that I have not been able to do because of drinking.”

Oscar declared, “Like last weekend in the Big Apple?”

“You got me there. But I’m referring to big picture goals like career, marriage, and living quarters.”

With a rising voice through the word, Oscar asked, “Marriage?”

“O.K. Strike that example.”

Oscar jumped on that last gaff by asking, “Has your drinking affected your relationships?”

“My drinking did not help in my first marriage. There’s no question about that. But it is also pertinent to note that Martha was mentally ill. Specifically, she had and still has an untreated, and in my estimation severe, bipolar disorder.”

“It’s interesting how every alcoholic’s ex seems to have a severe psychiatric disorder.”

“I can assure you that in my case it is well documented.

“Let me make another point if I may Oscar. The hard-core types are going to drink regardless of the circumstances. A friend of mine did that. Rocco, a traveling salesman drank cheap rot straight out of the bottle which I find crass. Rocco didn't like bars; he drank alone in fleabag motels. He only goal was to get totally fucked up. Now imagine if you will someone sitting on the edge of a bed getting plastered alone, passing out in his clothes, and pissing his pants. How utterly sad. I never pissed my pants in my life!"

Oscar quickly responded, "The final result is the same: gross intoxication. And I'll bet Rocco was at a significantly lower risk of certain complications by staying in-doors."

"You would lose that bet Oscar because Rocco died of upper gastrointestinal bleeding secondary to cirrhosis. He hit it hard on a daily basis. Listen, unlike me, he had no interest in bar room merriment and meeting interesting people. His only objective was to get as drunk as possible alone like the vast majority of alcoholics. That's not me."

Oscar slowly said, "Sounds sad either way. Gross intoxication is not a good place to be regardless of location."

I was exhausted. "Isn't there something in your AA book about bleating deacons?"

Oscar's deadpan look was his only response.

"The objective for me is to get feeling good but not falling down drunk, avoid blackouts, and do everything possible to make it through the spree relatively unscathed."

Oscar observed, "Collateral damage. Relatively unscathed. You talk like you are engaging in combat. Actually that's not far off now that I think about it."

"Let's face it Oscar; it is a dangerous world out there."

"Made exceedingly more so by your drunken adventures. I'm also beginning to get the picture that dangerous and bizarre episodes are part of the attraction. You like telling your drunken stories. You enjoy the laughter even though the only one laughing is you. And you like living on the edge."

"What's wrong with a little laughter and excitement?"

"Muggings, waking up in strange places; don't you see in all of these stories that you are powerless over alcohol and that your life is unmanageable?"

"Sure. But I'm not always powerless, and I mange my life pretty well when I'm not drinking thank-you very much, which is far more often than not. That is, most of the time I'm not even drinking let alone drunk. Broad brush Oscar. Let go of the broad brush."

"Would you agree that you cannot reasonably predict what will happen when you pick up that first drink?"

"Brother are you ever redundant. But sure, my New York City story is a good illustration of that. Once I start drinking, without sufficient safeguards in place, especially my big man, I can end up almost anywhere. But I need to keep coming back to the same point. Wouldn't you agree that, with all else being equal, a guy who gets drunk every day is 13 times more likely to get into trouble as someone who gets plastered only once every two weeks? And is it really your conclusion that the wisdom I have from advancing age, my many experiences, and my insisting on having certain safeguards in place before I walk out the door will have no effect on lowering the risk of collateral damage?"

"All the other things are not equal Freddie. A daily housebound drunk only goes back and forth to the liquor store. You are all over the map. Frankly, I think your drinking pattern or more precisely your behavior when you drink, puts you at a higher risk for something catastrophic to happen."

"That's the problem with AA's, you can't be objective. Everything is extreme. 'Oh, oh, you're going to end up in prison. Oh my God, you are going to die or be put in a mental institution. I love the last one; they don't even put street psychotics in nut houses anymore. But AA's keep saying it. Drunks are everywhere but in a mental hospital."

"Quite frankly Freddie, you are headed for something horrific. And in all my experience as a recovering alcoholic and counselor, I have never seen such extreme denial and rationalization."

"Look Oscar, I'm not denying that I'm an alcoholic. I was born an alcoholic. But when you factor in everything I have been talking about, I can make a credible case that I can drink relatively safely."

"Wow!"

"Wow what?"

"How's this. Based upon the history you have provided; your drinking keeps putting you in very high-risk situations. Alcoholism is a progressive disease and in your case it has progressed significantly. Every time you drink you are playing Russian roulette. Alcoholism is a bio-psycho-social disease and you hit on all three cylinders: family history of alcoholism, low self-esteem, and growing up in Buffalo where one's social life revolves around the tavern. You hit the trifecta."

"My self-esteem is not that low."

"We'll resume next Thursday."

"One more thing Oscar. I honestly believe that food is more of a problem for me than alcohol. Every time I lose weight, and it is an unbelievable struggle that takes both dieting and working out to do it, I relax a bit and boom, the weight is right back like some horrible recurrent disease. I'm more likely to drop dead of a heart attack than anything connected to booze. I'm in good shape now, but when the fat returns as it always does, I would be willing to take my chances with Ebola to halt this recurrent scourge."

"You will have to talk about your eating disorder with someone else. Ebola you say? Somehow that doesn't surprise me. You're a real pip Freddie."

Driving home, I concluded that Round II was close, but I gave myself the edge. And Oscar never acknowledged my most important point. I fantasize about wonderful things while in a zone of serenity: sophisticated cocktail lounges, great music, laughter, comradery, women … I could go on and on. These Walter Mitty-like daydreams sustain me, feed my spirit, and stack up pretty good when I consider the ratio: pleasant daily musings about my next drinking episode; romanticizing the drink if you will, divided by unpleasant drunks after the window of tranquility closes and slipping into a blackout. Being objective, I also factored in shaky mornings.

The calculation was stunningly in my favor. I couldn't wait to share it with Oscar. I knew I would blow him out of the water in Round Three.

***

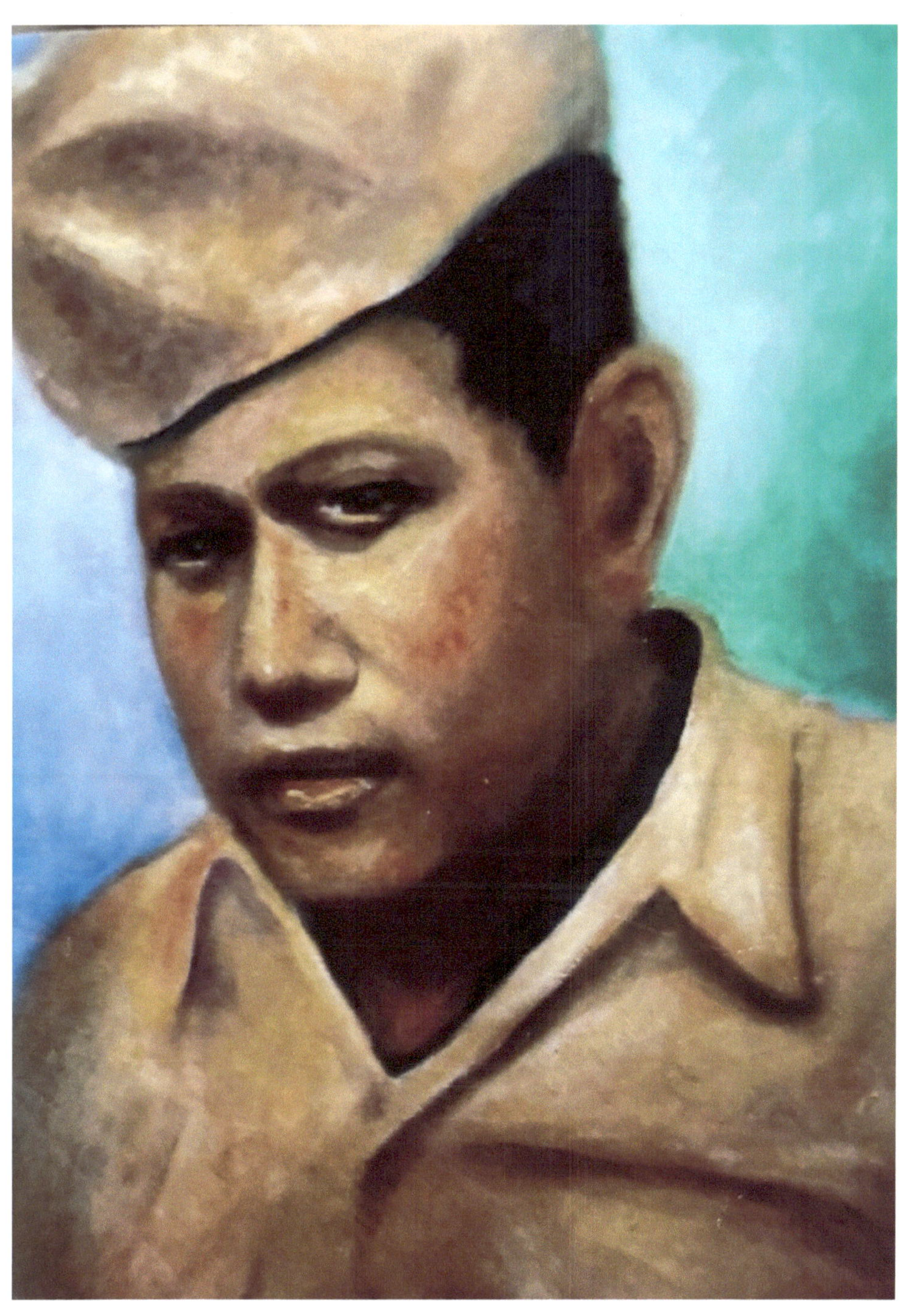

Carlos
KIA, WW II
NYC VA Regional Office Museum

Freddie and Oscar: Round III

I arrived for my next appointment in black tuxedo pants, a white dinner jacket with a pink carnation in the lapel, a black shirt with French cuffs, a black bow tie, and black patent leather tuxedo shoes. The recently bought white dinner jacket was very expensive, but I had a critical point to make.

Oscar was wearing an unimpressive white, skin tight polo shirt. He slid his black-framed glasses on the tip of his nose. With caramel-colored eyes above his glasses, he looked me up and down and scoffed, "A little over dressed are we today Freddie?"

Still standing, I replied, "Just making a point. I'm a long way from being the street alcoholic you are trying to make me out to be."

Oscar cleared his throat and with hoarseness still in his voice asked, "Please sit-down Freddie. I want to move on to another area that, based on what you have stated thus far, has been adversely affected by your drinking. Specifically, did your drinking cause problems with your first marriage that ended in a divorce?"

"I thought we covered this. As I already told you, Martha has a severe bipolar disorder. And oh, by the way, the marriage ended in sobriety. I hadn't drunk for almost three weeks before she walked out. But yes, my drinking contributed to some of the problems. I thought we had a reasonable solution near the beginning of the end."

"A deal for you to keep drinking?"

"You could call it that. While living in D.C., Martha lowered the boom by demanding, "You have to do three things or leave. Number one, go back to AA; number two, see a psychiatrist; and number three, fly to Buffalo every couple of months. She thought I must be drinking to excess because I missed my family. I can't stand my family. But my immediate thought was hallelujah; I couldn't have come up with a better plan."

"Why?"

"I believed then that Buffalo was the answer to all my problems—a nice three-day weekend drunk every couple of months with no one to hassle me about it. Flying back and forth with no driving or wife to worry about; that's all the time I needed. I was never close to being a daily drinker. And it was something to look forward to; a reason to carry on quite frankly."

"How did that work out?"

"Not so great the first time around, but this was due entirely to my not having a sedative."

"Again?"

"Yes. But that is only the 4th or 5th—no more than the 4th time actually—in recent years. It was President's Day weekend, and I went up to Buffalo for a three-day bender under her plan, and after—"

"Her plan absent the alcohol. What happened in 200 words or less?"

"I came back on a plane after 3 days of heavy drinking. I didn't want to drink that 4th day returning home, but I had the shakes bad. It gets harder to taper off with booze alone after more than a couple of nights drinking. The binge lasted 10 days. I have the image of trying to ride a bucking bronco. That binge culminated in that 9-day detox hospitalization I referred to in our first session."

"Let's pause here Freddie and focus on what you just said. Your drinking adversely affected your marriage and job, and you ended up on a 10-day binge which necessitated a 9-day hospitalization. That's two days over what normally is the maximum detox stay because of severe alcohol withdrawal. Didn't you say you had DT's during that hospitalization?"

"Full blown. I almost died."

"Well?"

"Well what?"

"You just said you had DTs and almost died! You mean to tell me that you don't think that is diagnostic of severe alcoholism?"

"It is if you look at it in isolation, but I would have never kept drinking like that if I had a sedative or if I was home alone. My wife locked me out of our house. I could have tapered off with booze in my own bed. And with or without Martha, if I had had a sedative, I would have been back at work Monday morning fresh as a daisy."

"Fresh as a daisy?"

"No. To be honest, I would have been a bit shaky but functional."

"And drinking while sitting in a bathroom stall again. When did you go to AA?"

"My first AA meeting was in the summer of 2002 after an isolated, single night of drinking, albeit it was a nasty episode. I'm sure I didn't plan to drink that evening as I had to work the next day, but while walking toward the subway, I turned left instead of right and found myself sitting at the bar in the Fox and Hounds British Café in the middle of happy hour. I didn't normally slip up during the workweek out of fear I wouldn't make it in the next day. I called my wife a couple of hours later and lied, 'Honey, I'm stuck with some people from work, including my boss. We are brainstorming about an important project that—' She hung up on me. I guess I had used that excuse one time too many. I must have thought since I was screwed anyway, I might as well make the most of it."

Oscar rudely interrupted, "That and the craving kicking in. Trying to stop after that first drink is like a weekend golfer hitting a 250-yard drive straight down the first fairway and saying, 'I think that's enough for me today.' "

"Such hyperbole Oscar! I happen to play golf. Ridiculous."

"As I was saying, I woke up at the Mayflower Hotel with a basket of fruit and a bottle of wine that had only one gulp left in it. I was still in my suit and tie, but my watch and the money in my wallet were gone. My wallet was on the floor; my credit cards were in it, along with everything else except my money. I had a vague recollection of a woman being in the room, but I had no idea where I met her. I was extremely nervous and the little bit of wine did nothing to calm my shakes. I had no desire for any of the fruit, although it was an impressive display."

"At the Mayflower? I'll bet it was."

"I was in trouble. I called my wife and she hung up again. Then I called my boss and lied about being sick. Actually, I was sick, but I obviously couldn't tell him I was in alcohol withdrawal. I told him I had the runs."

"Lovely."

"Ahem. I called AA next and was told there was a noon meeting at Saint Matthews's church a couple of blocks away. I went to the hotel bar and had a couple of drinks using a credit card before walking the few blocks to the church."

"That was nice of the prostitute to leave your credit cards."

"I didn't say anything about a prostitute. You really like to fill in the blanks to build a strong, one-sided case."

"If you are talking about alcoholism Freddie, you're the one building a strong case. You don't need my help."

"As I was saying, by the time I got to the AA meeting at noon, the expensive but pitifully weak drinks had worn off and I was violently shaking. I shared something—a cry for help I suppose. I'm sure they could hear the tremor in my voice. People came up to me after the meeting, and I ended up with a lot of business cards with phone numbers. Within a week I threw the cards out as they were unnecessary remembrances of horrors past. My thinking then and now is that ending up in AA means the bottom of the barrel, the gathering of the bums, the end of the line. I have known many drunks a lot worse off than me."

"Worse than you? If that's where you were drawing the line, that is a very low bar indeed. But returning to the Mayflower incident, you have identified another consequence of alcoholic drinking."

"Like what?"

"You're ending up with a prostitute. That and being robbed, which apparently is a common complication of your drinking."

"Not all that common when you consider how often I was drunk over a span of so many years. That kind of thing, losing a lot of money, only happened a handful of times. So, if we are talking percentages, I would say that over my entire drinking career, the frequency of getting robbed or losing valuable things is under 10 percent."

Oscar interjected, "And we are only talking about losing money and things of value, one of many complications of your drinking."

"Let's put it this way Oscar. I can accurately say that I did not have any serious problems more than 50 percent of the time, and I am older and wiser now. As to the Mayflower Incident as you put it, please drop the word prostitute. I don't know who the woman was. My best guess is I met her at a bar and asked her up to my room for a drink, as evidenced by the bottle of wine. Since it was empty, we must have both had a few. I also woke up with my suit and tie on; she certainly didn't dress me. Besides, and you won't believe this, sex was probably the furthest thing from my mind because I was married and drunk. I think I invited her to my room for a drink and passed out. How could I have known she was a thief?"

"Fully dressed absent your watch; a strange woman in your room; on the outs with your wife; missing work; little memory of the night before; losing all your money; a night at the Mayflower with that basket of fruit with wine, which must have cost a pretty penny; and in acute alcohol withdrawal. That's quite a list for one night."

"I already pointed all of that out. We are talking about rare occurrences that yes, are due to getting drunk. I'm being completely honest, which is more than I can say for your typical drunk. Alcoholics are notorious liars."

"It sounds to me that you have to tell a whopper on occasion?"

"Not that often. I wouldn't lie at all if it wasn't for my wife and job."

"You would not have to lie at all but for the drinking. You would have nothing to cover up. It's actually a great feeling."

"Not as good as those first few drinks Oscar."

"Oh yeah. That window of tranquility. Too bad it slams shut Freddie. The high is rather fleeting isn't it, always followed by deeper lows."

"Always? There you go again."

I added, with great emphasis, "And another thing. AA's don't seem to distinguish between a guy that is usually sober with infrequent bouts of intoxication from a lush that gets plastered on a daily basis!"

Oscar barked, "You keep making the same lame point. We don't call those in-between periods sobriety."

"We don't? Whose we? I'm not part of any we."

Oscar sat back in his chair and calmly lectured, "They are what we AA's call dry drunks. Much more often than not, these dry periods in-between drinking episodes are marked by irritability and an obsession about drinking—we call it the caged animal syndrome—until the inevitable happens."

"I already told you I like thinking about the next drunk. Using your golf metaphor, it's like fantasizing about a subpar round with a string of birdies."

Oscar ignored my excellent analogy and pontificated, "This is all characteristic of severe alcoholism Freddie. You are one of the worse cases I've interviewed."

"Come on Oscar. What about all the derelicts stumbling around in the streets? I'm sitting here in a tux!"

"So, you want to stay on the elevator until you get to the bottom floor? Alcoholism is a progressive disease. It always gets worse; never better."

"I must reject your absolutes: always this, never that. Life is a bit more nuanced my friend. And that includes drinkers like me."

"You're beautiful Freddie."

"Look, I wouldn't mind going to meetings if they didn't have this rigid, unrealistic demand of complete abstinence for the rest of your life. Meetings for periodic drinkers like me would be great if we discussed strategies for reducing the risk of unpleasant consequences of one's drinking. It would also be nice if modern medicine could come up with a pill to lower one's risk. There needs to be a more realistic approach to functional, borderline alcoholics like myself."

"A pill?"

"That's right. Antabuse has been around for a long time. If you drink on top of it, you become violently ill and usually end up in an emergency room. I ought to know because it happened to me. I was seen in an outpatient clinic after a head injury and stupidly took an Antabuse pill some nurse gave me. I waited more than 24 hours to drink, but I still had what I thought was a heart attack and ended up in a hospital ER. I thought I was going to die."

"You have to wait 72 hours. I'm sure whoever prescribed Antabuse told you that."

"I don't remember. Why can't they develop a pill that doesn't kick in until the 4th or 5th drink? Or better yet, after the 10th drink? If we can go to the moon—"

"And you would have had that 11th drink, but not the twelfth because you would be on your way to an ER."

"Not necessarily. By the way, something weird happened after that first AA meeting."

"Oh? Pray tell."

"I wish you would drop the Shakespeare. I used to get panic attacks well beyond any expected period of alcohol withdrawal because of my PTSD. I ran into a woman from that first meeting. We passed each other on the street downtown—I had already walked around the block several times trying to shake off this panic attack—and we recognized each other. Standing on a busy sidewalk, I launched into a tirade about panic attacks with fear that I was going to fall into a psychotic abyss. I remember saying, "I'm supposed to be at work; I've been walking all over downtown, circling blocks. I feel like I am on the edge of going stark raving mad."

The woman, short with curly red hair and freckles, said, "Oh. Yes. I had one of those last week. Right now, I'm thinking of killing myself."

I answered, "I understand. I've been there. Why just the other day I wanted to jump off the Peace Bridge."

After an uncomfortable period of silence, we simultaneously looked at our watches and I said, "Have a nice day" before we went on our separate ways.

Oscar stood up, slid his glasses back over his eyes, and spouted, "Alcoholism is a disease that is manifested by physical, mental, and spiritual sickness. The Big Book describes alcoholism quite succinctly: a physical allergy and a mental obsession in need of a spiritual solution. And it is a progressive disease, a point confirmed by the American Medical Association and the American Psychiatric Association, among many other relevant, prestigious scientific groups world-wide."

"So, you told me already. Everything is black and white. I think you're brainwashed. You and your ilk remind me of the classic cult film Invasion of the Body Snatchers, walking zombie-like, mindlessly mouthing your clichés, trying to pull anyone who drinks into your cult."

"Your ilk?"

"You heard me right. You AAs are all alike. You sit around in your parallel universe, with little contact with the outside world—the real world. In such a state, you are constitutionally incapable of acknowledging that guys like me can pick and choose our spots."

Oscar responded, "Can't you see that you are totally obsessed with drinking? You can't turn off such an obsession. Alcoholics are selfish and self-absorbed to the extreme. Booze is #1, even at the expense of loved ones like a spouse and children. It eventually controls much of your life, and I'm including dry drunks."

"If it ever gets to that point Oscar, I would voluntarily check into a 28-day program and go to AA on a daily basis."

"Look Fred, when it comes to matters pertaining to whether we should drink or not, active alcoholics are insane. You are having a conversation with yourself, an alcoholic, about whether you can drink safely. It's like talking to a crazy person."

Undeterred, Oscar continued, "And these escapades you have described; it's as if you are bragging. Do these drunken episodes make you feel more alive?"

"You mean did they?" I suppose. But I'm much older and wiser now. I actually have a healthy fear of walking on the wild side. There are benefits to aging."

"You are 40 Freddie; not in your 60s or 70s. More importantly, my sense is you are more careful when not under the influence. You are addicted to booze and where your drinking takes you. It's the chaos and extremely bizarre behavior that you see as comedy, whereas others see as sick and suicidal. And to say this can't happen again is not consistent with what you said earlier. You said, when I'm drunk, I—"

"When I was young Oscar. There's a song by the Animals entitled, "When I Was Young." A line from that song is, 'Pain more pain but a laugh-a-much louder yeah, when I was young.' In other words, there was a time when I was willing to take my lumps for a good story. For example, when I was 18 and in Times Square with my buddy Bum O'Brady—"

"Bum?"

"Yeah. Bum. His nickname. Why?"

"Nothing. Go ahead Freddie. Tell me what you did in the Big Apple with Bum."

"We were both 18, and I talked him into going to New York. We were in Times Square drinking at the bar in a fancy Chinese restaurant, The House of Chan. On my way out I took a statue of Buddha from the lobby. Two Chinese guys chased me down the street. With some considerable twisting and foul language back and forth, they finally got the Buddha and roughed me up pretty good in the process. Bum's looking at me lying on the sidewalk saying, 'What the fuck Freddie?'"

Oscar interjected, "Looking at you on the sidewalk roughed up, Bum was saying, 'This is why you dragged me to New York?'"

"Exactly. That Buddha statue was awfully big."

"And the point of your story is?"

"I had a lot of abrasions from hitting the sidewalk—some very painful, including black cinders imbedded into the skin on my knees because the falls and dragging along the sidewalk caused rips of my pants over the knees—but we eventually had a lot of laughs about that episode when I was young. You can get a lot of mileage out of an episode like that. But there's no fucking way I'm going to do stupid shit like that at my age."

"Are you sure about that?"

"Positive. I'll give you another example."

"Another drunk story. Oh joy."

"When I came back from the Persian Gulf, I was arrested in a motel room for being drunk and disorderly. They handcuffed me in my bathrobe and socks and hauled my ass to jail. I ended up sleeping in a bull pen with a bunch of druggies and drunks. I took off and rolled up one of my socks to use as a pillow. I appeared the next morning before a judge in my bathrobe wearing one sock pulled up to my knee. I pulled the edges of the bathrobe together, holding on for dear life as I was nude under the robe."

"O.K. Freddie, let's stop right there. Why did you add the part about the robe and sock? Like the Buddha statue. You like the comic element to the story. You like telling it. You probably like some of the crazy stuff you don't remember fed back to you. This is a part of your addiction"

"So? What's your point Oscar?"

"It couldn't be any more obvious. But let's just stick to the drinking. You see Freddie; you are on a course to end up as a lonely, pathetic figure that will die an ugly premature death. I'll tell you something else. Somehow—by luck or grace—you have avoided the catastrophic. But your luck is going to run out."

"There was another incident in New York with a woman I met in a bar who had a very strange skin disease."

"Stop it! Let's pull the plug on this. Skin disease. Jesus Christ!

I didn't like Oscar's abrupt way of ending the session, so I slammed the door on my way out. But I had to, begrudgingly, give him the edge on Round III.

***

Freddie and Oscar: Round IV

While Oscar had the skin tight black polo shirt on again, his muscles and tattoos were not the least bit Intimidating. However, he stood behind his desk and did not shake my extended hand; rather, he folded his arms and said, "I'm afraid we—"

Suspecting I might be getting the hook while still being in hot water with my wife—I welcomed a divorce but not as the result of my drinking—I interrupted with, "Let me say at the outset Oscar, that I finally see your point about the progressive nature of alcoholism and I have begun going to AA meetings."

Sitting down and inviting me to do the same, Oscar answered, "I'm glad to hear that Freddie, but in order to get much out of AA, you have to stop drinking. Incidentally, vodka does have an odor to it."

"I can't smell it."

"I smell it now. It's coming out of your pores. There is a distinct smell to old vodka and it's not pleasant. You reek of it. How often are you going to AA meetings?"

"Every day", I lied. "But I can't say I like them. By the way, I wonder whether there is such a thing as odorless alcohol? You would think with all the advances in medicine there would be."

Oscar stood up again and folded his arms, which I thought was odd as I just got there. Looking down at me, he declared, "You are at a critical crossroads Freddie. One path leads to a sober, relatively happy, and productive life. The other road leads to more suffering, chaos, and eventually premature death, prison, or an insane asylum. For many alcoholics, such a choice is difficult to make."

"Of course, it's a difficult choice. I have met some miserable AAs and a lot of happy drunks. Also, as I keep saying, drunks do not go to insane asylums. Jails and the morgue yes, but let's drop the nut house shall we. That's another AA canard."

"I'll use your language Freddie. We are talking about percentages. Do you honestly think an active alcoholic has a better chance at a serene life than a sober one working the program of Alcoholics Anonymous?"

"If you are talking about this alcoholic Oscar, the answer is yes. Absolutely. I feel a lot better drinking in a nice lounge on a Friday night after a hard weeks' work rather than sitting in some musty smelling church basement watching assholes beating their breast or preening about the room because they haven't had a drink for X number of years. Big fucking deal. The world doesn't give a shit if Joe Blow didn't have a drink today. Besides, just having the option to drink gives me considerable peace of mind. To be perfectly honest, I don't give a damn about how other alcoholics feel, drunk or sober. This is all about me."

Oscar said, "That's one thing we can agree on."

"There is something else to keep in mind Freddie. Many people a lot wiser than me have said the alcoholic stops growing emotionally when he begins his alcoholic drinking."

"That's absurd. That would make me 12 years old. My history—and I have been very frank about it unlike your typical drunk—shows that the steady downward spiral of progression is a lot of bunk."

"Bunk? Millions of people in AA can give witness to this, including many physicians. It is well documented in the medical literature. Bunk you say?"

"That's right, as it applies to me. To me Oscar. It's rubbish."

Looking bewildered, Oscar sat down and said, "You're a real piece of work."

"One other thing Oscar. Would you be willing to be my sponsor?"

"No."

"No? I thought that you guys can't say no."

"That's generally true but in your case Fred, there's no fuckin way."

"Freddie."

"We are finished here. However, I can recommend someone to you. Aengus McCarthy. He's better known as Whitey."

"Whitey?"

"That's right. Whitey. Here's his cell number. Call him between 10 and 11 pm tonight; he'll be home from his meeting by then. I'll give him a heads up. He never refuses a call for help."

"Thanks a lot Oscar," I bitterly said through clenched teeth.

I walked out and threw Whitey's number in the trash. Nevertheless, as there were no points to add up for Round Four, I was victorious: 2-1.

***

Alone

My wife Nicki asked me to leave because I was not staying sober as promised. While she denied it, I knew she had talked to Oscar. I felt violated. But I offered no protest. On the contrary, while I walked out the door with my head hanging low as I knew Niki was watching me, once I was in my car, I was singing the Animals' song "It's my Life" (and I'll do what I want).

A week later, on my 41st birthday, I found a furnished apartment. No more nagging. No more counselors. I pulled into my new parking lot with stuff loaded in the trunk and back seat, got out, and did the Irish Jig, overflowing with gratitude.

I went out drinking that night to celebrate. I went to a nice restaurant with what I remembered had a lively happy hour crowd in their small cocktail lounge. I was in there once with Niki; while having dinner that evening, I kept eyeing the busy bar. I heard the loud laughter, music, and the tinkling sound of the ice hitting the glass—the enticing song of the Sirens—but with Niki virtually keeping me tied to the mast, I felt like the caged animal that Oscar referred to. But on this night, breaking the bondage of marriage, finally liberated, I went back seeking fellowship with kindred spirits.

Sitting at the bar in the Persian Palace, trying to look at myself in the mirror and only seeing a blurry image, I looked to my right and left. The bar was empty. (That kind of thing seemed to happen all the time; I'd see this good looking, fun happy hour crowd when I couldn't join them because I was with my wife, and nothing but empty barstools when I had my opportunity. But it was all good; the field was perpetually clear.)

The bartender, a tall, thin, middle aged man with a neatly trimmed salt and pepper beard and mustache, probably noticing his customer's eyes were now three quarters shut as I asked for another drink, said in a Farsi accent, "I am sorry sir, but I cannot serve you."

"Why?"

"I think you are intoxicated."

"That's ridiculous. I'm tired more than drunk."

"Well sir, I—"

"That's all right. If you would be so kind as to call me a cab."

"Certainly sir. Right away."

I offered no further protest. On the contrary, I concurred with his judgment and appreciated the call for transportation, saying, "You're absolutely right. What I need is to get safely home and to bed."

The taxi dropped me off at a familiar haunt. I've been told many times that I look cock-eyed when drunk. But normally, if you can stay on your barstool, you'll get a drink at the Blarney Stone. Besides, it was dark with a good-sized crowd. Nevertheless, I only showed the bartender the left side of my face as I ordered a drink, followed by a further turn of my head away from him while yelling, "Hey Billie!" to no one in particular. The old buzzard served me two drinks before shutting me off. Pretending you are recognizing someone in the crowd will work once, maybe twice, but never thrice. It's pretty embarrassing to get shut off at the Blarney Stone.

I blacked out. I probably took a cab home. It must have been a little after 4 am as that is when the bars close in Buffalo. I apparently collapsed on the couch with my clothes on. At least that is the way I found myself many hours later. It was not very often that I remembered anything past midnight let alone coming home, so there was nothing unusual up to this point, other than waking up at 1 pm, the first time I slept continuously that long in years. I must have taken my sedative in the middle of the night to get ahead of the withdrawal. I probably took a double dose. (I can relate to Michael Jackson in that and only that respect: lying in bed, tossing and turning, all I want is to be knocked out, not realizing that I already had enough in me to put down an elephant.)

After the 11 hours of uninterrupted sleep, I was quite nervous upon awakening as expected, so I took a double dose of Ativan. After two hours of additional rest, I took another double dose and started drinking, merely sipping at first, and I briefly felt like I was entering that temple of delight. I always have this desire—I know now it's a compulsion—to enhance the jag. But the enhancement is a blackout. Booze wasn't working for me. It never really did.

During the hour or so period of time that I was coherent, I made some phone calls to old drinking friends. I brought up tired old topics of drinking escapades with each friend, desperately trying to be funny, but falling flat. Every friend found an excuse to quickly terminate the call. I felt intense humiliation, but that faded fast with more alcohol.

However, the feeling of loneliness persisted. Sitting back on my dark brown fake leather couch with many cracks in the plastic, holding a tall glass full of bourbon over ice cubes looking at the bottle of Jack Daniels on a glass end table in front of me, I was crying and had no one to reach out to; at least no one that I wanted to connect with in the condition I was in. I ordered anther fifth of bourbon for delivery from a nearby liquor store and kept drinking.

My life was blank for several days thereafter.

***

The Hospital

Lying in my hospital bed in the intensive care unit (ICU) on the first morning of consciousness, a woman's voice coming through a white cloud hovering over me said that I had overdosed on drugs and alcohol and sustained a serious head injury. Groggy, I laid in bed looking at a ceiling fan go round and round, trying to remember what happened. The strained mental exercise was futile.

A physician explained that I had sustained a subdural hematoma and drugs had been administered to reduce brain swelling. He also raised the possibility of intracranial surgery. As he droned on, the gravity of what had happened did not completely escape me, but my predominant thought was I needed a drink. It became an obsession, expanding in my mind, pushing out all other thoughts and concerns, to include the pain I was inflicting on the dwindling few that still cared about me. I am certain that an alcoholic's brain chemistry changes when we are obsessing about drinking. It's like being on a run-a-way train barreling toward booze. There's no logic to it; there's no exit ramp. And the degree of anxiety was steadily rising as it always does with alcohol withdrawal. I knew sedatives were contraindicated with severe head trauma; accordingly, I had terrifying fears of hallucinations and seizures.

I can't remember if anyone explained why I didn't have the intracranial surgery—that's how battered and befuddled I was—but when I was moved out of the ICU, I distinctly remember Charge Nurse Jesse McColl. She was no nonsense, old school, and harsh. McColl was a very large woman with no neck—just the head with an angry face on broad shoulders—and she wore the traditional white dress, stockings, and cap even though it was no longer required, which I found exceedingly peculiar but was this a nightmare? Someone that fit that description definitely said "absolutely not" to my request for a sedative. I thought about leaving, but with tubes coming out of me and no clothes, that was not an option.

I had a grand mal seizure that evening, which medical staff attributed to my head injury, but I knew it was from alcohol withdrawal. Whether drug induced or from the seizure, I slept for many hours and at some point, I evidently signed a consent to be transferred to an alcohol treatment program.

***

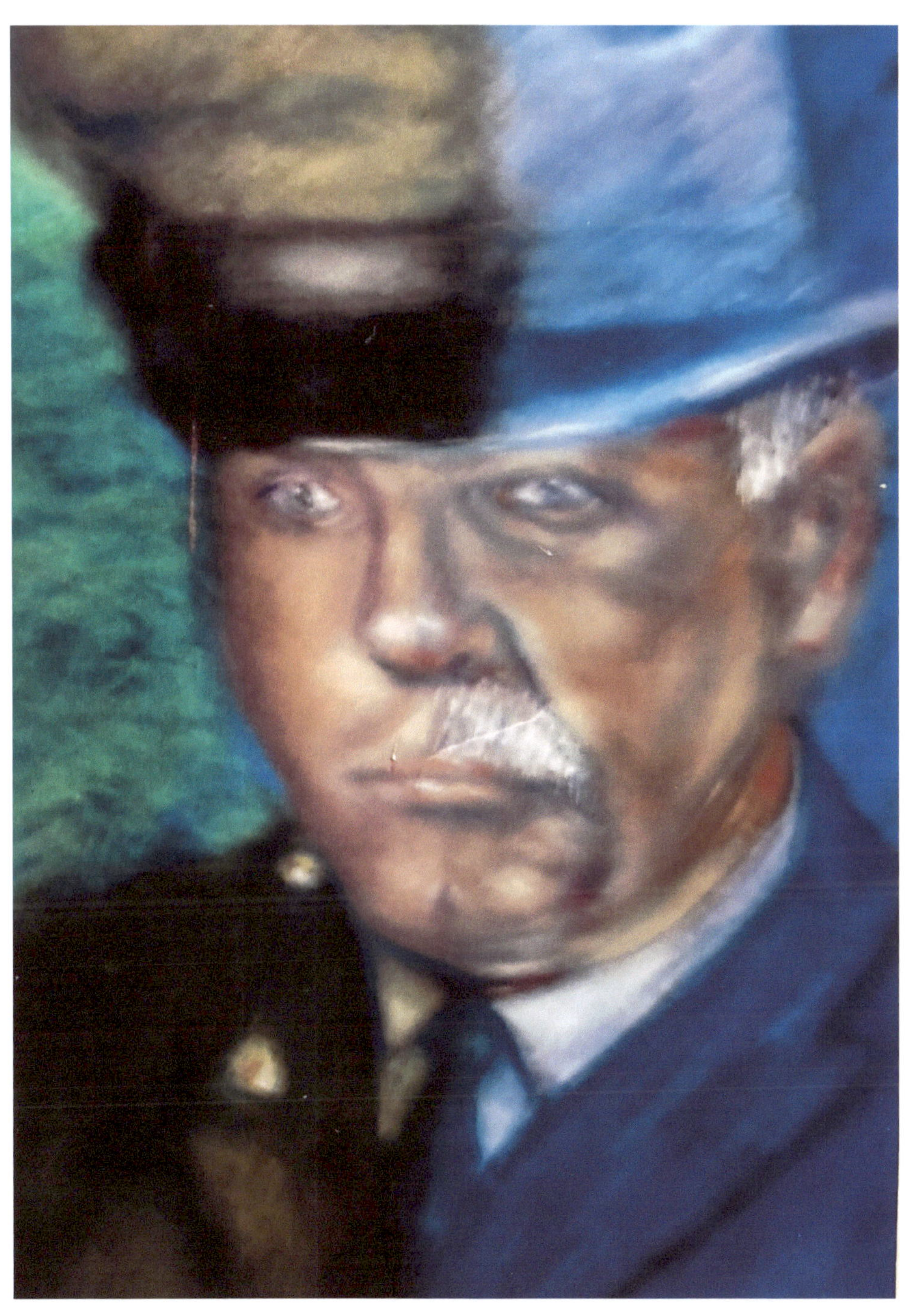

Rick Williams
(Self Portrait)
Vietnam

Rehab

I was brought to the admission room of the 28-day treatment program, We Are Not a Glum Lot on the morning of September 11, 2001. Upon arrival, I was crawling out of my skin. I was told that since Glum was an alcohol and drug treatment program and not a detox facility, sedation would not be administered.

Given the number of days that had elapsed since my last drink, the extreme anxiety was not booze withdrawal; it was an uninterrupted panic attack due to my understanding of the serious nature of my head injury, a long-lasting blackout of several days' duration without any indication of where I was, who I talked to, or what I did; and leaving another trail of alcohol-related mess behind me. My plots and plans and schemes of desperately trying to control my drinking were clearly not working, yet I saw no life possible without alcohol. It was not only being doomed to a life of boredom; I could not function in society without booze. More importantly, stripped of all defenses, to include rationalization, comedy, and lies; a devious, despicable degenerate was all that was left. I decided that the only way out of this terrifying nightmare was suicide; the only question was how.

I was still in my clothes and had my wallet before the admission procedure was completed, and with the entire staff occupied with something horrible that had happened in New York—I heard voices coming from CNN reporters and gasps of "Oh my God" from staff—I walked out of the hospital. Being an irrevocably broken basket case and humiliated beyond belief yet again, I felt driven to jump off the nearest bridge. Walking briskly through the parking lot with no idea of which way to turn, I hesitated. I don't know what made me look inside of a van with "We Are Not a Glum Lot" logo on both sides of the vehicle, but I did. The keys were in the van so off I went, finding a bar on the first corner I came to.

Sitting on a stool in "The Old Sod," the small TV was to my left, in a nook above the bar, and I listened to and watched the unfolding horror in lower Manhattan. I drank three shots of Jack Daniels in less than five minutes. The young bartender gave me a funny look after the third one, but I could not have cared less. Once steadied, I was ambivalent about taking my life at that moment; I became concerned about getting the stolen van back without being detected and what was happening in New York City and Washington, D.C.

***

Rock Bottom

I made a decision to return the vehicle after having one more drink. I was horrified by replays of the collapsing twin towers, 200 floors of steel with 3,000 people disintegrating into gigantic, billowing clouds of dust that burst through and ran down narrow streets enveloping stunned pedestrians trying to escape.

I'm not sure how many I ended up having, and I don't remember leaving, but it must have been the middle of the afternoon. The next thing I remember was hearing screams and feeling a warm burning liquid in my eyes. I couldn't move. I opened my eyes and saw a shadowy face looking down at me. I tried raising my right arm but couldn't. I asked, "Where am I?

The face behind a veil of fog with a soft dispassionate voice said, "You are in the intensive care unit at Erie Country Medical Center. Don't try and move. You sustained injuries to your head and spinal cord. A physician will be in soon to explain everything."

I tried to move my other arm. Then my feet. I couldn't move my arms or legs. "Am I paralyzed?"

The blurry image faded away, but I heard a muffled, "The doctor will explain your injuries."

"Was anyone else hurt?"

The nurse said, "I'll be back in a few minutes."

I remembered the screams. I did not feel any pain. I didn't feel anything but overwhelming, smothering fear.

I heard beats from a monitor. I turned my head to my left. There were a lot of tubes, some seemingly connected to me, but I couldn't feel them in my body. There were strong medicinal smells; I could also smell my perspiration.

I was short of breath and felt my heart pounding against my bones. I turned my head to find the same blurry face. She had no expression. I panted, "Did I hit someone?"

My eyes rolled back and to my left to watch the nurse injecting something in a hanging IV bottle. I could see her oriental eyes. She replied, "Someone will be in to talk to you about that."

Still breathless, I gasped, "Did I hit someone?"

This time her head didn't move; she raised her voice and said with contempt, "Yes. You hit a 12-year-old boy."

I cried out, "Dear God in heaven. Please. Please let the boy live. Take me. Please let it be me. Let me die. Take me."

With the bed raised 45 degrees, I could feel tears burning on my cheeks, but something stopped them from running down the right side of my face and there was a stinging sensation where they stopped. I couldn't touch my face. I couldn't touch anything. I felt moisture on my forehead. Things went blank again.

I heard talking. I opened my eyes and saw a shadowy face with a dark beard and black framed glasses state coldly, "My name is Dr. Edwards. You suffered a spinal cord injury."

"Am I paralyzed?"

"It is too soon to say. We need to further examine you and do some tests."

A nearby voice of a higher pitch and scornful tone said, "Let's not beat around the bush with this guy. It's all over the news anyway."

There was a terrifying pause.

With each word dripping with disdainful rage, the same person with the higher-pitched voice said, "Your spinal cord was severed. You are paralyzed from the neck down. That is for life; there is nothing anyone can do to change that. You drove off the road, into a grade school bus stop. The boy you hit is dead. He was 12. Your blood alcohol level was consistent with gross alcohol intoxication, four times the legal limit. Four times! Two young girls were also injured. You plowed right through them drunk. We do not know their condition since they were taken to another hospital. There are detectives waiting in the hallway to talk to you about it."

"I can't. No. Please."

"I'm sending them in."

There was one hazy face with a hat and two voices. The questions were like ice picks into my brain and chest and gut. I had no memory of the accident. Hyperventilating and light-headed, I was unable to speak. Accident? It was murder. I wanted one of them to put a slug in my temple. But the most appropriate punishment was for me to wake-up each day— incarcerated—with the knowledge of what I did and my paralysis from the neck down greeting me as soon as I opened my eyes and staying with me every waking minute of the day.

I never saw my wife Niki again. From where I lay now that marriage looks like heaven. She was intelligent and compassionate. I could visualize her momentarily, petit with her long auburn hair falling on her shoulders and big, dark, exotic Persian eyes. I had it all; much more than I deserved. Combing through cocktail lounges; crawling through dives; what in the name of God was I wildly searching for? I couldn't possibly find anything half as good as I already had. I'm not just referring to my wife; I'm talking about a life. But that was on paper. I was in the grips of an obsession that precluded happiness. Being an alcoholic was not my fault; refusing to get help was. Oscar offered his firm outstretched hand ...

The only thing Niki gave me a hard time about was my drinking. I remembered her looking down at me as I lay on the couch with facial abrasions from a fall, drunk, with her shaking her head in bewilderment. "Why? Why are you throwing everything away? All those years in school? You have worked so hard to get where you are. Our marriage? Your daughter? Why throw it all away?"

Why indeed.

That was a few years ago. I didn't have an answer for Niki's question. I do now. I was totally self-absorbed; a pitiful egomaniac with an inferiority complex; dishonest to the core; unwilling to accept the obvious and consider the help that was in front of my nose; running, hiding; a coward, afraid to off myself and spare the children that I killed and maimed and those that loved me—my mother—unrelenting shame.

My mother and daughter visited me in the hospital. My mother's eyes were ringed with red and full of tears. Her voice repeatedly cracked; I couldn't understand her. My daughter looked at me deadpan and said, "I don't feel sorry for you. I don't feel anything except disgust."

Choking on anguish, I stammered, "I'm sorry" and turned my head away from them.

Oscar visited me in the hospital. I almost didn't recognize him in a charcoal grey suit and black turtleneck sweater. He was brief and spared me the I told you so's. He left AA cassettes and a tape player. Whispering, I asked him if there was any way he could sneak in a lethal dose of a drug. He shook his head no saying, "You could be of service to countless alcoholics and addicts." After a pause, he added, "After all that has happened, you still don't get it Fred. Listen to the tapes." He turned and walked out of my life.

There was a trial. It went in painfully slow motion for a week. I was in a motorized wheel chair. An indistinct face sat atop a black robe. The jury and prosecuting attorney's faces were shimmering as if they were under a hot sun.

The jury returned their verdicts in less than 3 hours. I was found guilty on all counts, to include negligent homicide. I murdered a 12-year-old boy and destroyed a young girl's life.

And the families; there are no words to sufficiently express the outrage and pain of losing a child caused by a drunk's contempt for everything other than his twisted, sick wants and needs.

At the sentencing part of the trial, the parents of the boy I killed spoke. The mother, a petite woman with a pale face and curly brown hair said through halting sobs between every short sentence, "You killed our only child. He had many friends. Tommy was an excellent student. He loved his Mom and Dad. He loved animals. Tommy wanted to be a veterinarian. He was precious."

She paused and swallowed and looked up at the ceiling. Thereafter, shaking, she raised her voice and cried out, "I cannot describe the level of pain I constantly feel. You drank yourself into a stupor and got behind the wheel of a van without regard for anyone. You drove drunk in broad daylight when children were being released from school and ran over them. You sit here in your wheelchair and expect sympathy, but you will get none from me. You killed our boy and shattered our lives. Being in prison will not be enough punishment as far as I'm concerned." Life without my—" The mother broke down sobbing. She was helped back to her seat by her husband.

The father, with a contorted face of torment intertwined with rage, was large and well-built with piercing dark eyes. He spoke at greater length with rising anger. At one point he shouted, "I want to rip you apart with my bare hands." I bowed my head. He closed with, "I hope you burn in hell for eternity."

Every word of both parents hit my forehead like a hammer; I blinked with each blow. Oscar was right. Even at this point, after all the pain I caused others, my primary concern was me.

Gagging on every word, my mother spoke with frequent pauses to try and compose herself about my being an altar boy, a boy scout, and soldier in the National Guard in Desert Storm. She said I was never the same when I came home but that was not true; I was a supply sergeant and drank excessively before the service. I had begged her not to; it was the most painful part of the trial for me. She stumbled and fell getting out of the witness chair. My lawyer helped her stand and guided her back to her seat; she was sobbing and sniffling and moaning loudly.

I asked my daughter not to testify and she honored that request. My wife did not offer to.

I also tried to speak at the sentencing hearing, but not in the hope for a lighter sentence. I apologized to the family of the boy I killed. The boy I murdered. Apology? What an outrageously inadequate word. The tears were real, but they were for me as much as the family of the dead boy.

"I first want to express my deepest sympathy for—" There was dead silence in the courtroom. "If I could change places—"

The parents looked away. I stopped talking.

The girls I hit survived. One 10-year-old, Kelly, had a fracture in her left upper arm but recovered. But the other girl, Shannon, age 12, sustained multiple fractures in the arms, legs, and pelvis. Her recovery has been marked by surgeries, including a hip replacement at age 13; she loved soccer but will never play sports again. She faces more surgeries, ongoing physical therapy, and constant pain. Shannon will walk with a limp the rest of her life. There will be another trial, possibly two, and they will wheel me into the courtroom to face the children and more outraged parents.

I will always be in prison, mentally as much as physically. I am awake in a never-ending nightmare. Outside the walls, if I had the money and means, I would stay on morphine or better yet overdose on it. Serene nothingness. Still thinking of me to the bitter end.

During one of our last sessions, Oscar said that if I did the things that are suggested in AA, in earnest, I would change, become less selfish. He talked about a spiritual awakening and that rarely people fail that thoroughly follow the program. He also spoke of 12 promises. Serenity was one. I looked for serenity in a bottle and found eternal hell.

Oscar also read a quote to me from his AA book: "Contempt prior to investigation will keep a man in everlasting ignorance." Because of my contempt and selfishness, I murdered a 12-year-old boy, and severely and permanently injured a 12-year-old girl.

I was sentenced to seven years in prison. To be precise, seven years in a New York State Prison with a hospital. I am a quadriplegic. That means paralyzed from the neck down. I was able to hear from a television in an adjoining room that the parents and most of the community were outraged at the leniency of the sentence.

Nurse's aides turn me on my side several times daily to change my sheets, bathe me, take off my diaper, and wipe my ass. I don't feel anything when I defecate. There is no warning, but I smell it. I hear grumbled obscenities and feel my head thrust back and forth when the orderlies change my large diaper and sheets. My urine goes from my penis through a tube into a bag that is emptied three times a day. I can't feel the catheter, but I can smell the urine. I smell my own disgusting piss, shit, and sweat. They feed me through tubes. While I don't feel physical pain below the neck, I have daily headaches that are severe in nature. They refuse to give me anything stronger than Tylenol. But it is the mental torment that is never-ending torture. They won't medicate me for that either.

I had choices. Suicide can be painless and make sense for people like me—a walking, driving, ticking time bomb. Vacillation was my tragic flaw. And Oscar presented another alternative. He said with great confidence based upon many years of experience on both sides of the desk that a content life with periods of joy and serenity was virtually guaranteed. But I scoffed and dismissed all of that. I did it my way. I never gave AA a chance.

I listened to all of the cassette tapes that Oscar left for me. One of the speakers read the 12 promises of which Oscar spoke. If we are painstaking about this phase of our development, we will be amazed before we are half way through. We are going to know a new freedom and a new happiness. We will not forget the past or wish to close the door on it. We will comprehend the word serenity and we will know peace. No matter how far down the scale we have gone, we will see how our experience can benefit others. That feeling of usefulness and self-pity will disappear. We will lose interest in selfish things and gain interest in our fellows. Self-seeking will slip away. Our whole attitude and outlook upon life will change. Fear of people and of economic insecurity will leave us. We will intuitively know how handle situations which used to baffle us. We will suddenly realize that God is doing for us what we could not do for ourselves.

Where was God when that little boy's life was extinguished?

What did Oscar mean about me still not getting it? I get it. It's agonizingly obvious that I should have followed his suggestions: I killed a boy; ruined another child's life; caused immeasurable, never ending pain for the parents and my mother; and threw away my life in the worst possible way. But what does he want me to do? Get someone to wheel me into an AA meeting to give them my experience, strength, and hope? I have no hope. I have no future. It's about what could have been. No dead boy. No badly broken girl. No paralysis. And a life worth living. Instead, I am in prison on day # 36 with 2,521 days to go, about 240,000 excruciating minutes to endure, to think about what I have done. That's the only thing I can do. I can't shut my mind off. Tic, tic, tic. Think, think, think.

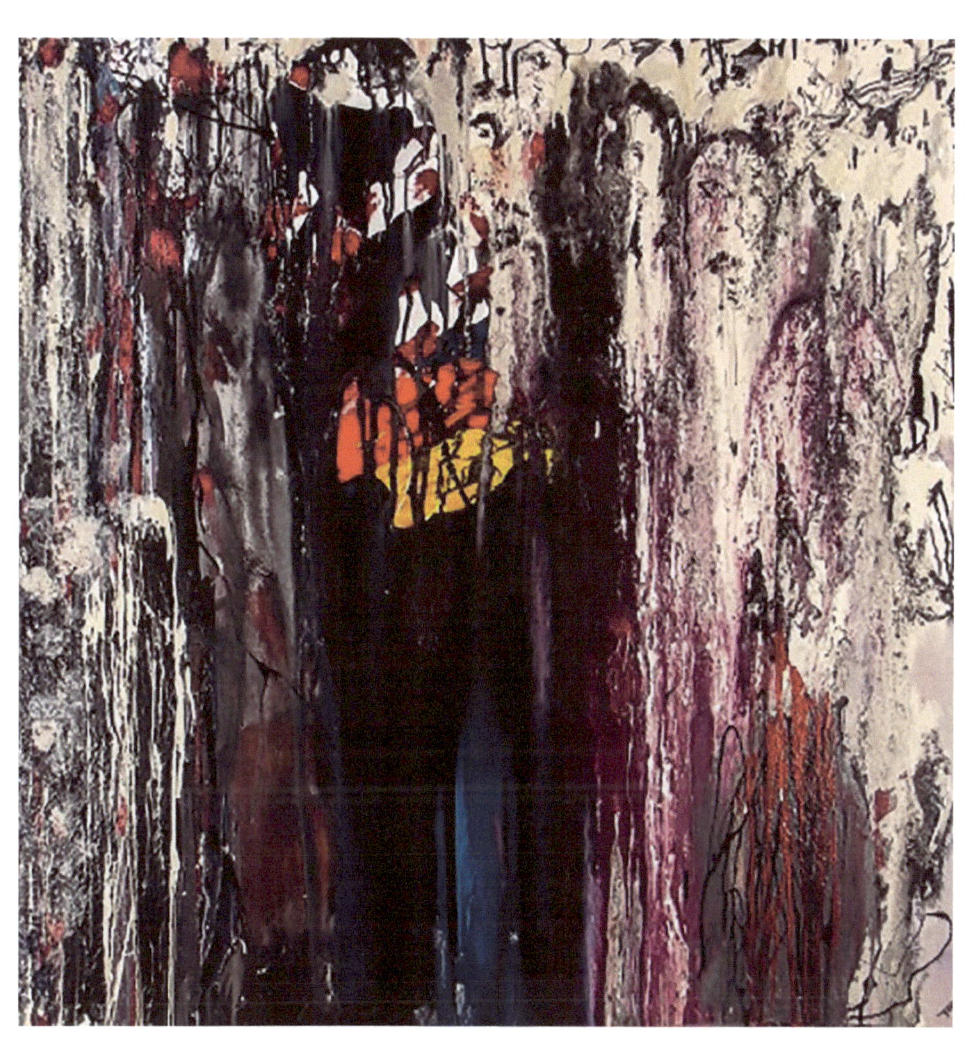

Hue 1968
The Inferno

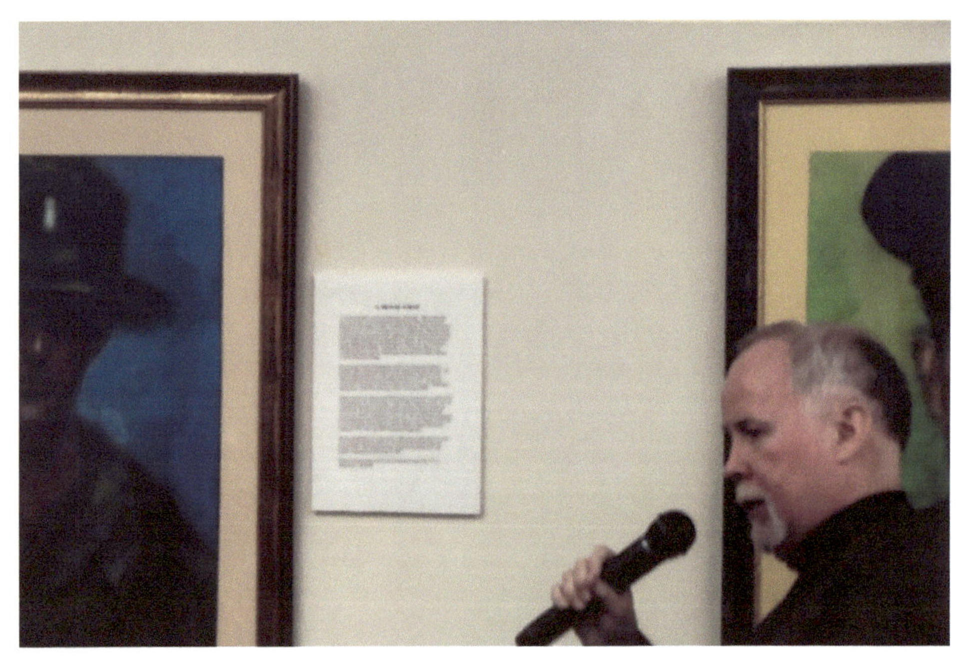

**"Twelve Veterans and their Stories"
exhibit held at the
NYC VA Regional Office Museum
in November 2006**

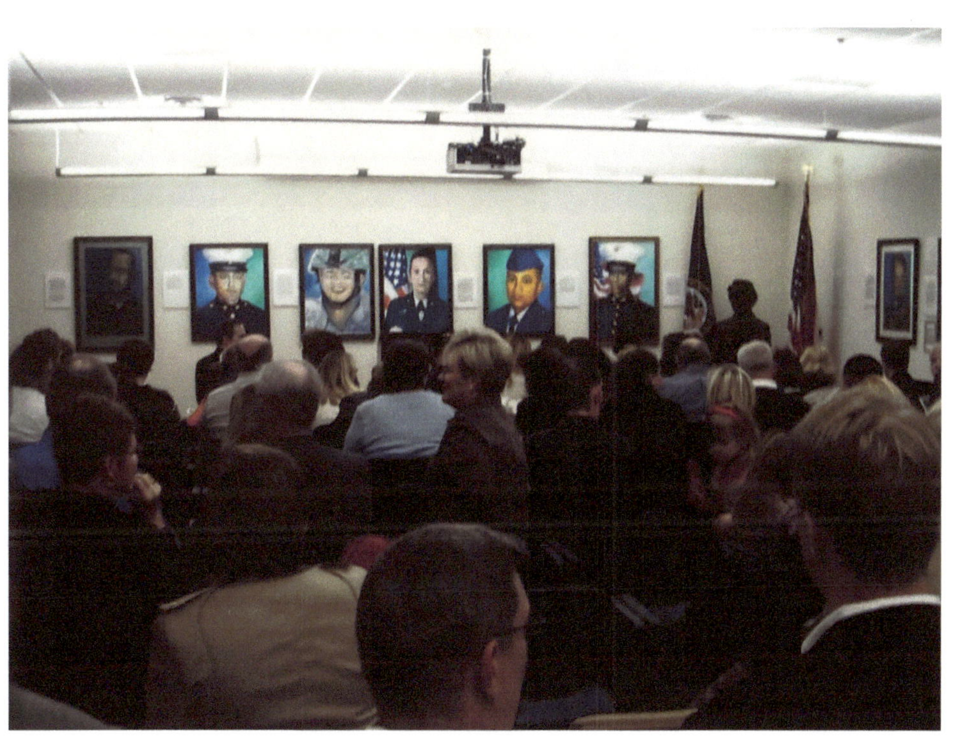

"Honor, Valor, Sacrifice, Service"
exhibit held in
Buffalo VA Regional Office
in June 2007